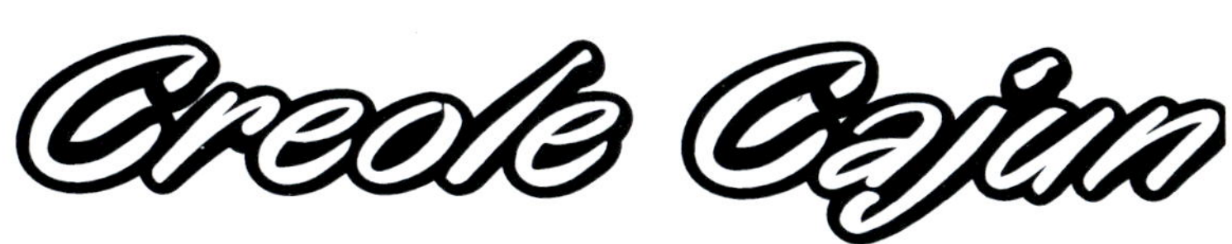

presents

Roux, Roots, & Recipes

New Orleans soulfood flavors that would wake up your ancestors

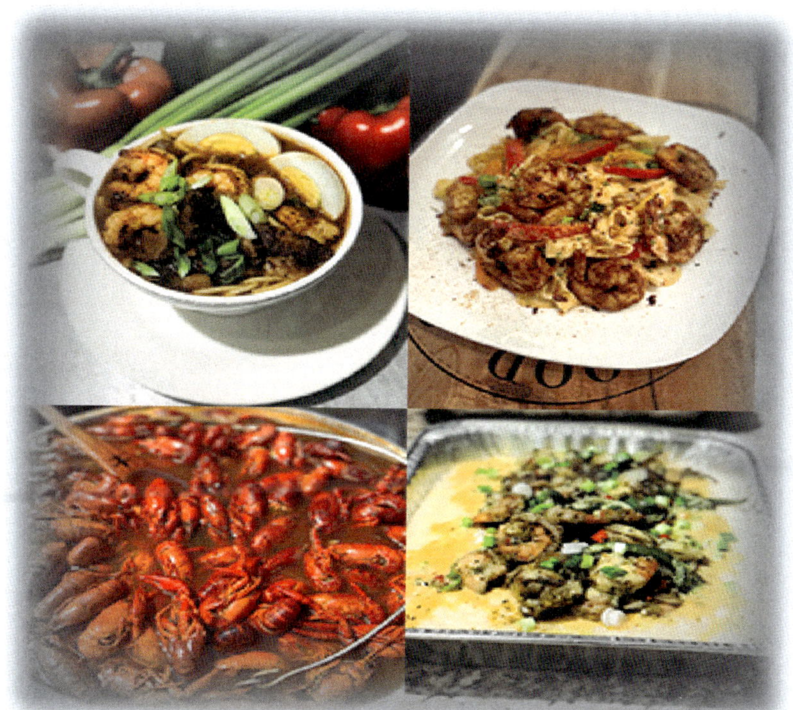

Gale Levy Boudreaux

Copyright page

Printed in
The United States of America

Creole Cajun Queen
Roux's, Roots, Recipes

Book cover, Graphics and Formatting by Butterfly Grafix
www.butterflygrafix.com

ISBN: 979-8-9851690-0-3

Table of Contents

Dedication

I would like to dedicate this book to my mom Barbara Levy, my father Lloyd Bridgewater Sr., my aunts, my sisters and brothers my kids Bryson, Toni, and Khalil my cousins and friends who inspired my memories, being my taste testers as I invoke on this journey. My cookbook is a personal expression of the love and joy involved in keeping families, friends and others together. I have learned from everyone on this journey. Knowing what flavors and seasonings each one of you likes, loves and lusts for has helped me to craft, create and cook foods that everyone enjoys.

Keep Cooking Sha' 🧡

5 Food Swaps

Creole Cajun Cuisine is rich in spices and seasonings. Also it relies heavily on shellfish and other meats. There are many lovers of this cuisine that have preferences and sensitivities that require substitute ingredients.

Below are my top five food swaps

1. *Replace chicken for the seafood*

2. *If it's too spicy leave it out!*

3. *Don't like meat baby throw in your bell peppers and onions. Keep the sauce!*

4. *If you want to cut the grease on your roux just make it dry.*

5. *Never leave your trinity out! (Bell Pepper, onions and celery)*

Shrimp, Sausage and Chicken Jambalaya

Oh it's carnival time! The smell of Jambalaya reminds me of Mardi Gras and my favorite fun Aunt Audrey. When she would come to visit us, she would sneak and dump my mom's milk out of the gallon carton and fill it with beer, LOL. Then she would watch my mom cook Jambalaya, as we had hot dogs and sodas to go.

Jambalaya has entered the American lexicon of cooking just based on the name. Yet its fame is no equal to the taste of this dish prepared right and served hot and fresh. Too be honest, once you've tried it fixed the Creole Cajun Queen way, you just might be so jaded you will never want the commercial version again. This is a dish you literally have put your foot, toes and ankles in. Everyone that's eaten it swears by it.

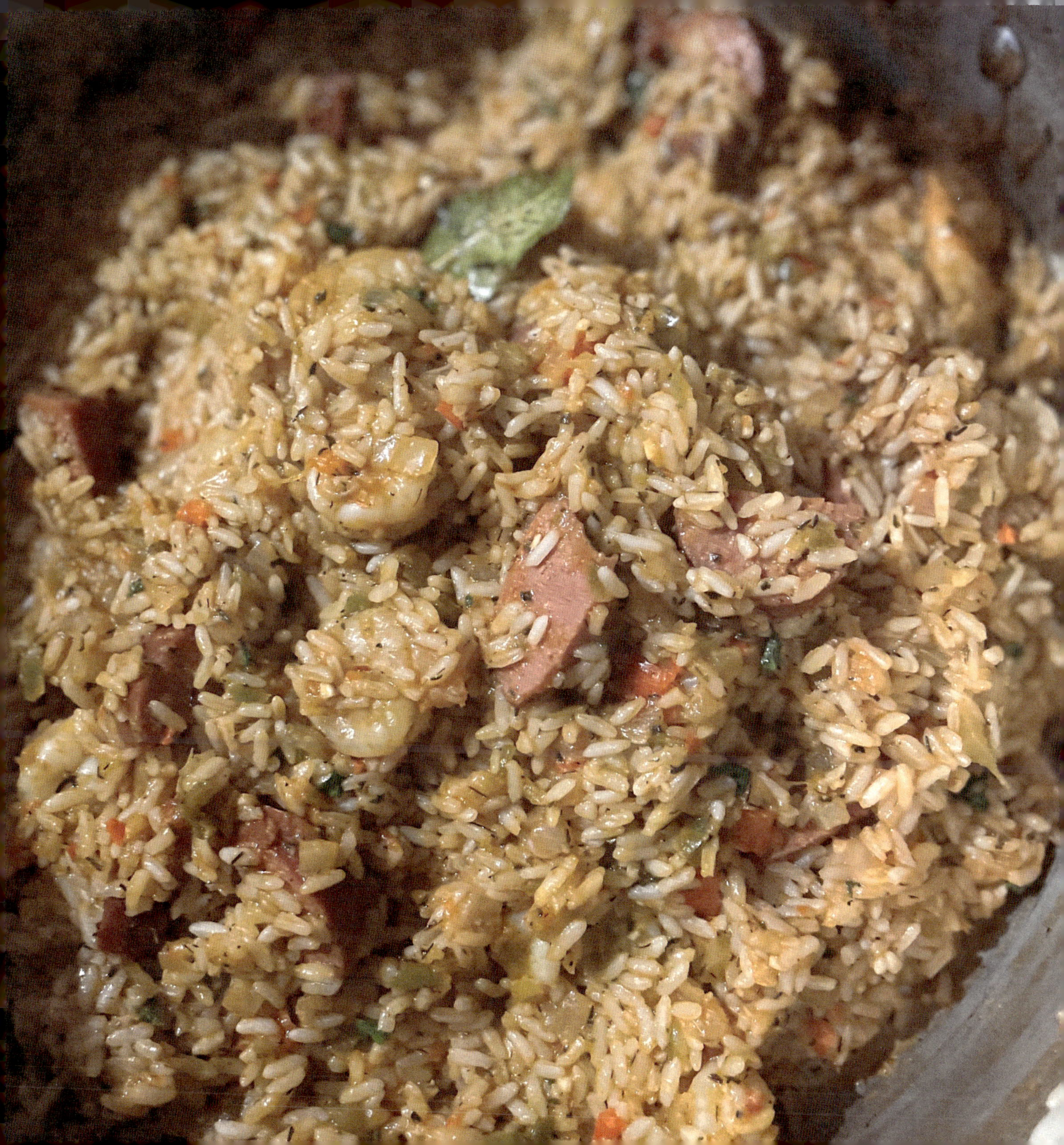

Ingredients

Serves 4-6

2 cups of long grain rice
1 lb. peeled , clean and deveined shrimp
1 chicken breast diced
1 lb. D&D smoke sausage
1 yellow onion
1 green bell pepper
1 Yellow bell pepper
1 red bell pepper
1 cup celery
1 cup green onions
1 tablespoon fresh Italian parsley
2 stick margarine
1 cup tomato sauce
1 cup chicken stock
1 teaspoon of Creole Cajun Queen creole seasoning *(use any creole seasoning or order mine on line)*
1 teaspoon thyme
1 teaspoon basil
1 tablespoon garlic powder
1 tablespoon onion powder
1/4 teaspoon crab boil
2 bay leaves
1/4 teaspoon salt
1/4 teaspoon black pepper
1 teaspoon white sugar

Instructions on next page

Instructions

1. Wash and cook your rice and set aside. Dice your onions, bell peppers and celery (trinity)

2. Slice your sausage, dice your chicken breast. In a cast iron skillet cook your chicken until internal temp is 165, then toss in your sliced sausage and shrimp Stir together on a medium heat... Keep your juices from the meat and set aside.

3. Add 2 stick of margarine to the cast iron with your trinity, salt, black pepper, basil, thyme, creole seasoning and sauté down on a medium heat until soft.

4. Add in the tomato sauce, chicken stock, crab boil, garlic powder, onion powder, bay leaves, sugar, add meats. Stir all ingredients bring to a simmer.

5. Cut your fire, add in your rice and mix evenly. Mix in your green onions and Italian parsley, plate and serve.

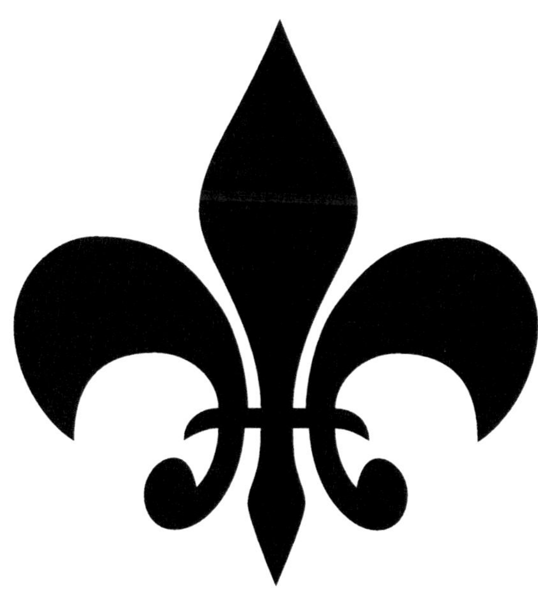

Creole Cajun Queen Smothered Corn Melissa

My smothered corn Melissa is an inspired friendship dish. Every evening after work before my little ones got home from school I would go over to my friend/ cousin Melissa's house and have gossip time over this favorite. I would always come around the time she is shucking her corn and boiling pickle meat (New Orleans salt meat) backed up with some good old kitchen conversation. Growing up, kitchen hopping in the neighborhood was traditional.

The secret ingredient is LOVE. As we hopped from kitchen to kitchen it was to experience the common elements of love and family. To hear the stories and to enjoy to feeling of community. Once the meal was ready and the friends were seated around the table that a shared meal was so soul satisfying. It was the result of preparation and participation and birthdays with friends also.

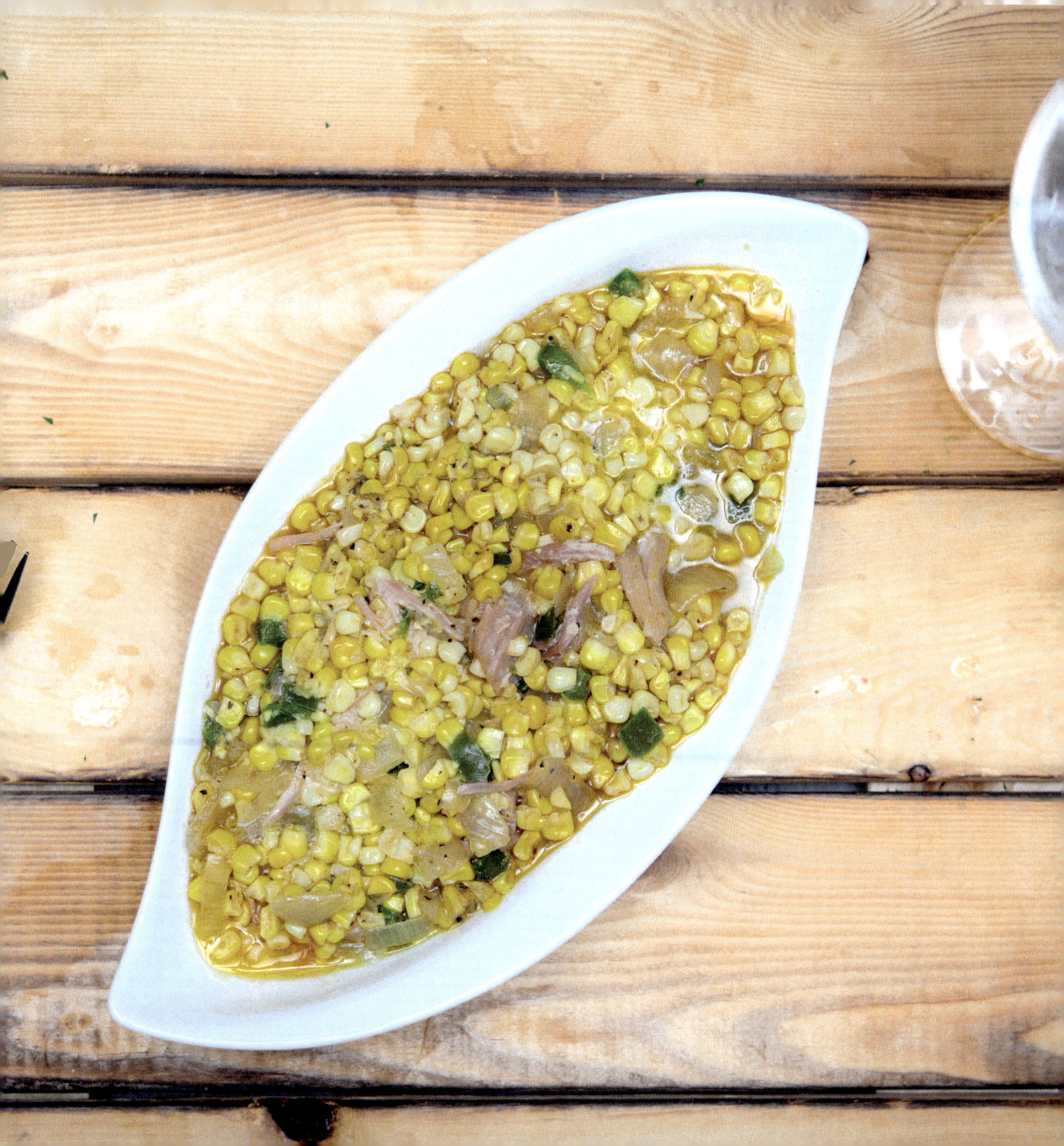

Ingredients

Serves 4-6

6 ears fresh corn
1 large yellow onion
1 green bell pepper
1lb pickled salt meat boiled or fried cook (ham optional)
2 cups white rice
1 stick of butter
1 tablespoon creole Cajun Queen creole seasoning *(use any creole seasoning or order mine on line)*
1 tablespoon onion powder
2 tablespoon bacon grease
1/2 teaspoon sugar
1/2 cup water

Instructions

1. First cut your corn off the cob in a bowl. Dice up your bell pepper and onions

2. Heat your butter and oil together in a cast iron skillet or metal pot on medium heat.

3. Once the oil is hot fry your corn getting it a little soft (10 minutes). Next add in your diced seasonings and toss/ fry together (10 minutes).

4. Add your meat then mix in evenly. Add all of your dry seasonings plus the sugar. Pour in a little over a 1/2 cup water, smother down enjoy the aroma and cover for 15 more minutes. You can serve this smothered goodness over rice and enjoy.

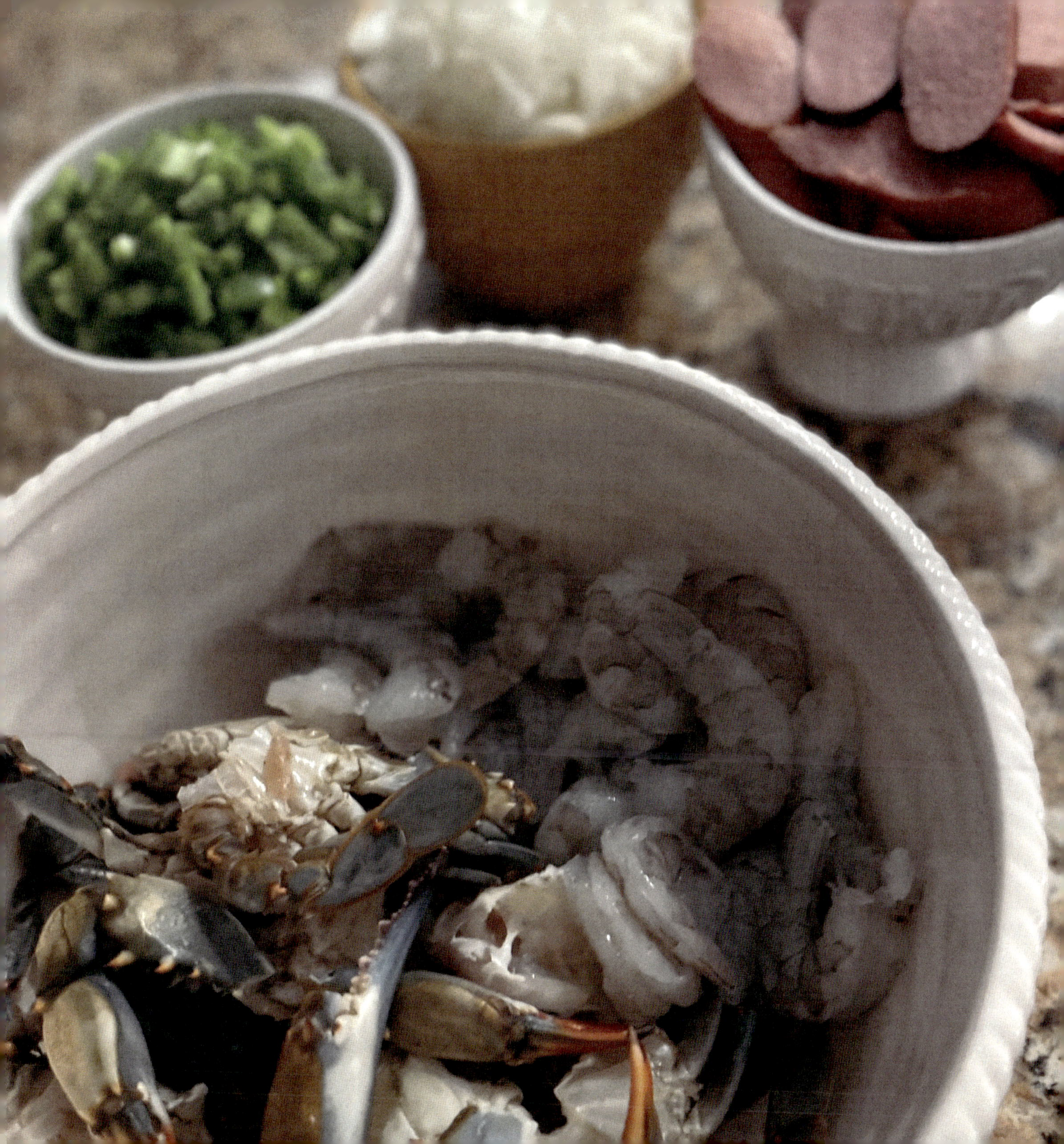

Creole Cajun Queen Shaka YakaYaka-Mein Soup

This soup brings me back to my club hopping days in New Orleans. If you are out at hole in the wall (neighborhood bar room) drinking with friends and you want to get up the next morning at 5 am for work straight and sober, then this is your soup.

A Spicy hot yet soothing broth (the hang over soup). This special recipe has also been known to help sooth common colds.

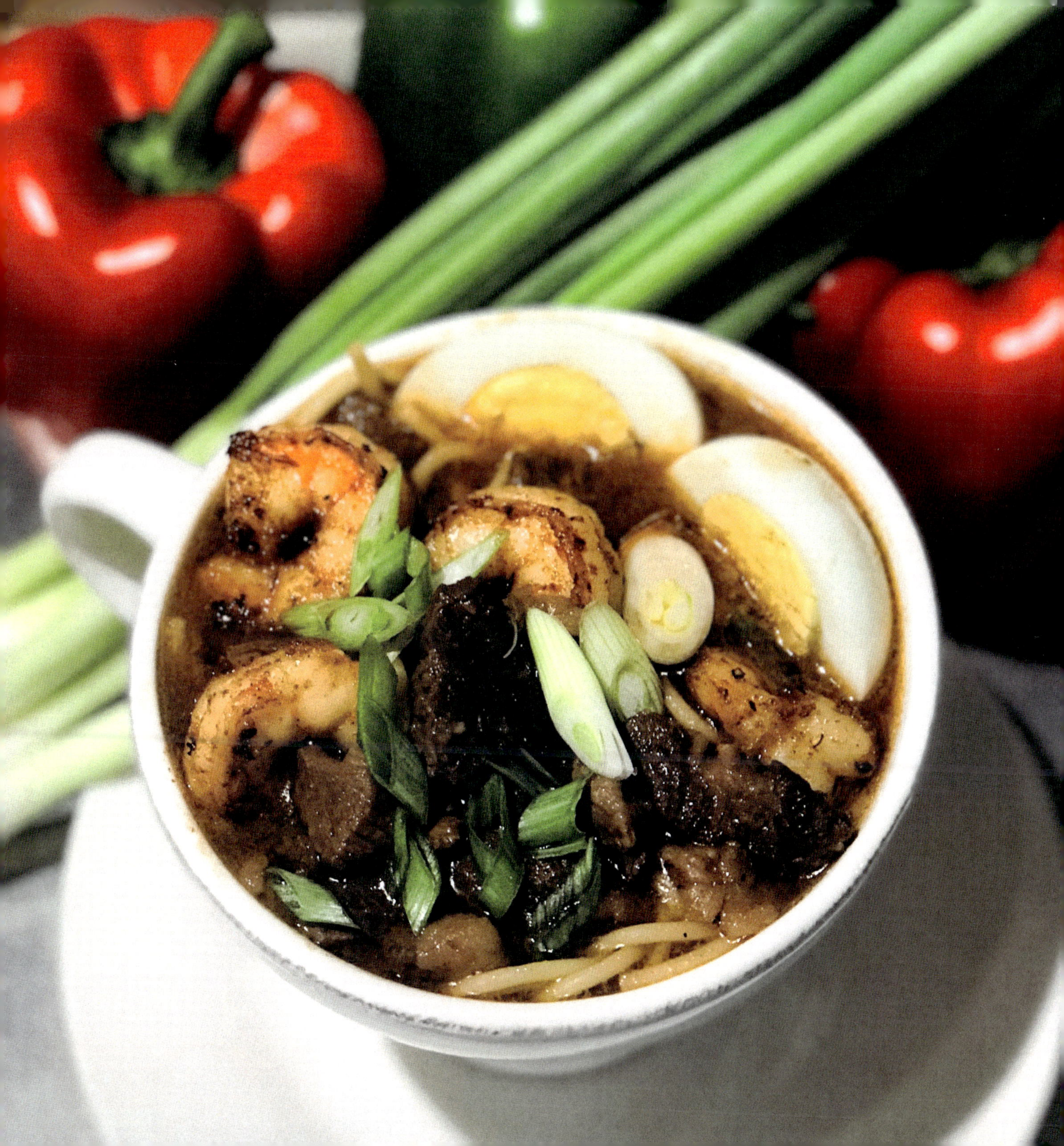

Ingredients

Serves 4-6

1 beef chuck roast(diced stew beef size)
1 lb. Deveined , peeled, Clean large shrimp
2-8oz can beef stock
3-cups of water
1 tablespoon chicken bouillon powder
1tablespoon beef bouillon powder
1 tablespoon black garlic powder (season for shrimp)
1 teaspoon cayenne pepper (I like mine a little spicy optional)
3 tablespoon garlic powder
1 tablespoon black pepper
1/2 teaspoon salt
1 tablespoon creole Cajun Queen creole seasoning *(use any creole seasoning or order mine on line)*
2 tablespoon onion powder
3 tablespoon soy sauce
1 tablespoon kitchen bouquet
4-6 boiled eggs (sliced)
1 8oz pack of linguine pasta (boiled)
1 bunch chopped green onions
3 tablespoon olive oil
1 dash of Louisiana Hot Sauce

Instructions

1. In a deep cast iron or metal pot heat your oil up to 350 on a medium heat. Season your diced beef with half of your dry seasonings. Fry your beef browning your meat all over evenly. Cover your pot. Juices from the meat will start simmering your meat.

(continued on next page)

Instructions (continued)

2. Keep your heat on medium and add in your beef stock, water, kitchen bouquet, chicken and beef bouillon, and your remaining dry seasonings to the pot.

3. Season and grill your shrimp in a separate pan and set aside. Bring your covered pot to a boil for 1-2 hours or until your beef is completely tender. Add in your grilled shrimp 30 minutes before finishing your yakamein.

4. Get your soup bowl layer it with your boiled pasta; ladle your shocka yaka soup covering pasta. Slice your boiled eggs place on top then garnish with plenty of green onions. Baaby serve and enjoy!

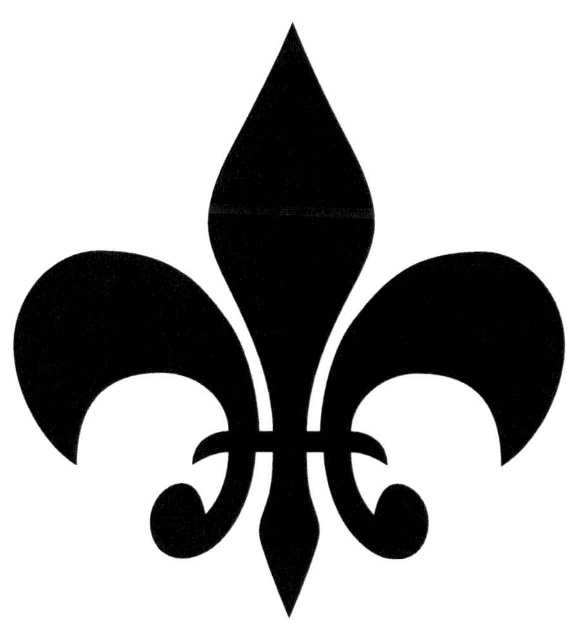

Creole Cajun Queen Southern Fried Catfish

Friday card parties, family arguing over spades and supper plates around the neighborhoods. Either you are fishing on the lake for your Friday catch or out enjoying fried fish at your mom and pop family restaurants. And yes I'm better in spades lol!

There was nothing like family and friends coming together to show who was the best spades player. Playing card games with and endless supply of fried catfish and all the fixing was not only sport...it was the essence of FAMILY! I can still taste the conversation an still savor the Catfish with everything that went with it.

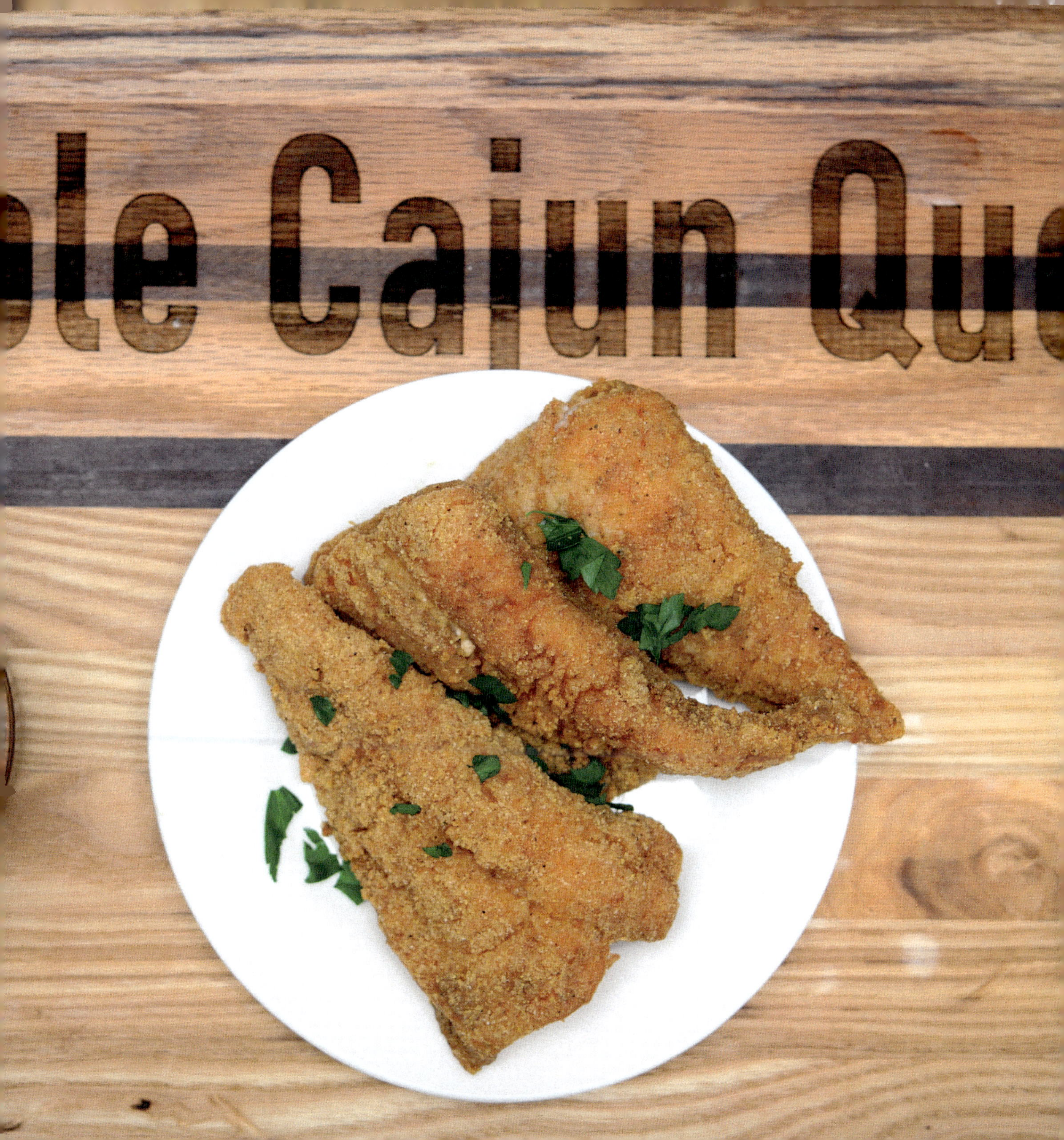
Cajun

Ingredients

Serves 4

4 fresh Catfish fillets
2 tablespoon yellow mustard
1 teaspoon black pepper
1/2 teaspoon salt
2 tablespoon black garlic powder
2 cups Seasoned lemon fish fry
1 cup yellow cornmeal
1qt cooking oil (your choice)

Instructions

1. Clean and pat dry your catfish fillets.

2. Season your fish with salt, black garlic powder and then gently rub your fish all over with the yellow mustard until evenly coated. Chill in fridge for 2 hours

3. Remove your fish from the fridge. You will need a cast iron skillet or a deep fryer. Heat your oil up to 350.

4. In a shallow square pan mix your seasoned fish fry and cornmeal together. Coat each piece of fish evenly shaking off Access fish fry.

5. Start laying your fish in the hot oil not moving them around as much for 7 minutes or until you see it float. Lift your fish, let it drain on a paper napkin and eat baby!

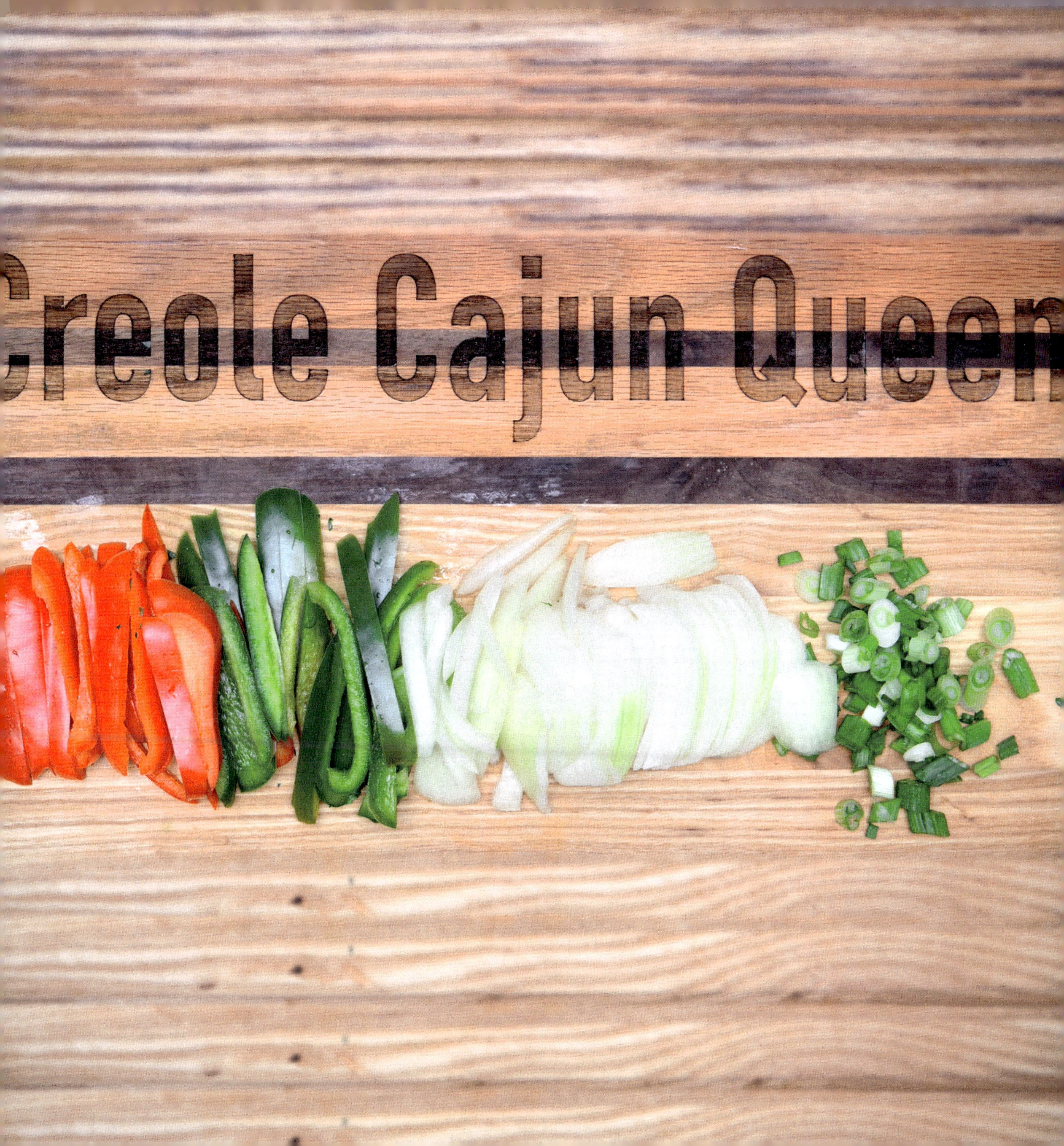
Creole Cajun Queen

7th Ward Stuffed Bell Peppers

I can smell Thanksgiving time when making stuffed bell peppers. Family and friends calling around the city to tell each other where the bell peppers are on sale. What store comes to my mind is Circle Food Store or the food truck that would ride through the neighborhood yelling on the loud speaker "Bell peppers! Creole tomatoes!!! It was like the Ice Cream Truck coming. I can still here neighbors screaming "Hold the Truck I'm coming!

Nothing said Special times better than savory stuffed Bell Peppers. They were part of the Trinity "Bell Peppers, Celery and Onions" My family would often say they would have to hurt you in order to pass along the secret of our Stuffed Bell Peppers. People would come from miles around to enjoy this delectable treat. Everyone would always ask for the recipe. (Now you got it) with everything that went with it.

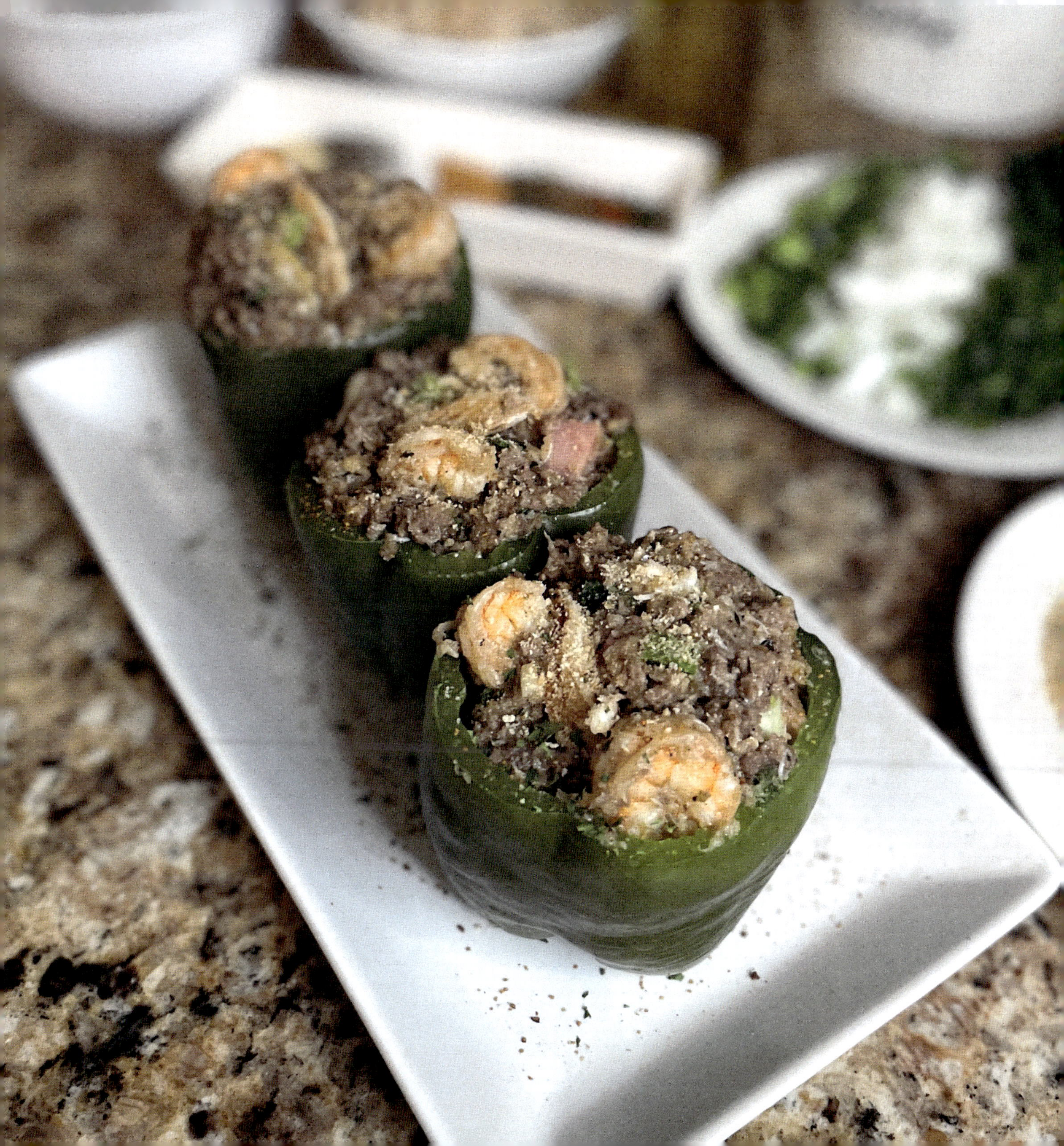

Ingredients

Serves 4-8

4 big green bell peppers
1 yellow onion
1 tablespoon chop garlic
2 tablespoon chop green bell pepper
1 lb. pork sausage
1 lb. ground beef
1 lb. peeled clean deveined shrimp
1lb lump crab meat
1 tablespoon Louisiana garlic boil boost
1 tablespoon Creole Cajun Queen Creole Seasoning *(use any creole seasoning or order mine on line)*
1/2 teaspoon crab boil
1 teaspoon thyme
1/2 teaspoon
1 tablespoon garlic powder
1/2 teaspoon basil
1/2 teaspoon salt
1 teaspoon black pepper
1 tablespoon onion powder
1 stick melted butter
2 cups Italian bread crumbs

Instructions

1. Wash cut bell peppers in half. Boil peppers until tender by firm and set aside, save 1 cup of the water for later.

(continued on next page)

Instructions (continued)

2. Clean peel and deveined shrimp. Save the shrimp heads. Boil shrimp heads in 1/2 tea spoon crab boil and set aside.

3. In a medium to large metal pot fully Brown the ground beef and pork sausage together and drain, transfer the meat back into your pot.

4. Stir in the chop seasoning, shrimp, crab meat and dry seasoning, mix together fully cooking the shrimp.

5. Turn off your fire, add your shrimp stock and saved bell pepper water stock gradually stirring in the Italian bread crumbs

6. Mix all together creating a stuffing/ dressing like mixture.

7. Stuff mixture into bell peppers, sprinkle with bread crumbs on top and coat with melted butter.

8. Bake for 30 minutes at 350 cool and serve.

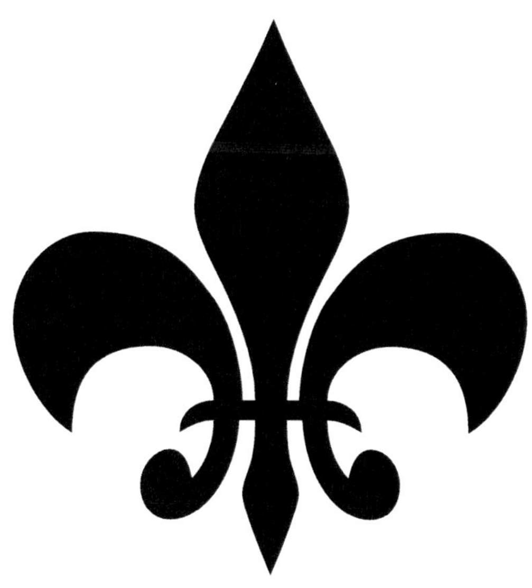

Creole Cajun Queen Shrimp & Steak Fried Rice

This fried rice is one of my hood mixed with Chinese recipe, lol One of my favorite Chinese restaurants in New Orleans inspired this recipe. I can also remember feeling like it was a special day when my mom would order there combination rice dinner. This rice brings me back to date nights, birthdays with friends also.

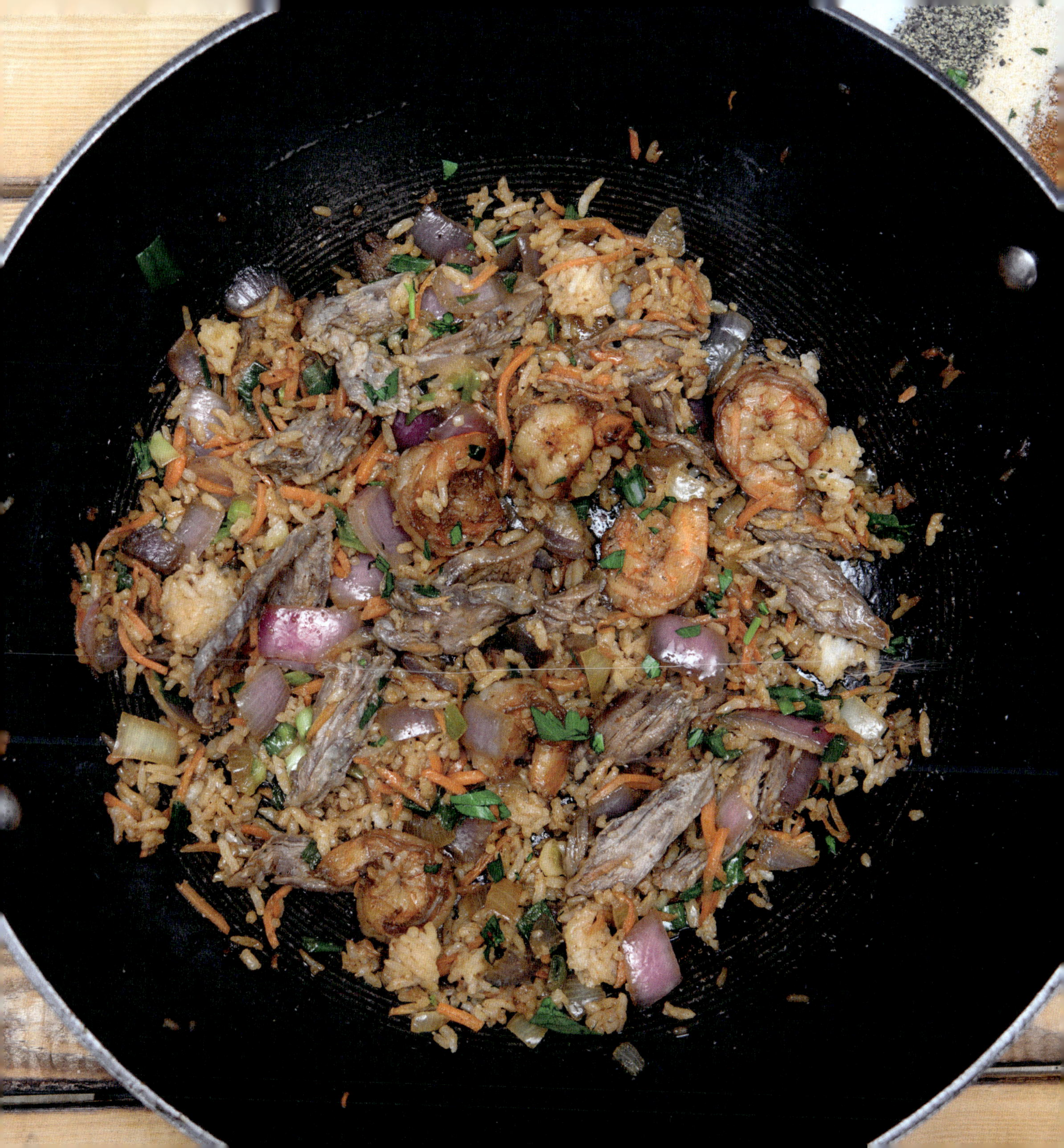

Ingredients

Serves 4:

1/2 lb. Flank steak (slice into thin strips)
1 lb. Jumbo deveined clean shrimp
2 cup cooked white rice
1/2 large diced purple onions
1 cup green onions
1/2 cup shredded carrots
1/2 cup sesame pure oil
1-2 tablespoon soy sauce
1 tablespoon garlic powder
1 tablespoon onion powder
1/2 teaspoon black pepper
A pinch cayenne pepper
A pinch Salt to taste
1/2 teaspoon black garlic powder

Instructions

1. Season your sliced flank steak and shrimp with black garlic powder, fry your steak first in sesame oil medium well then remove put to the side and then your shrimp. High heat watch oil

2. Keep sesame oil hot in the pan and start adding your purple onions, carrots, shred carrots, green onions. Fry down until soft.

3. Leave your fry going and add in your soy sauce mixing your cut seasonings together.

4. Cut your heat add in your steak, shrimp give it a toss; add your cooked rice, dry seasoning mixing together. Garnish with more green onion plate and serve.

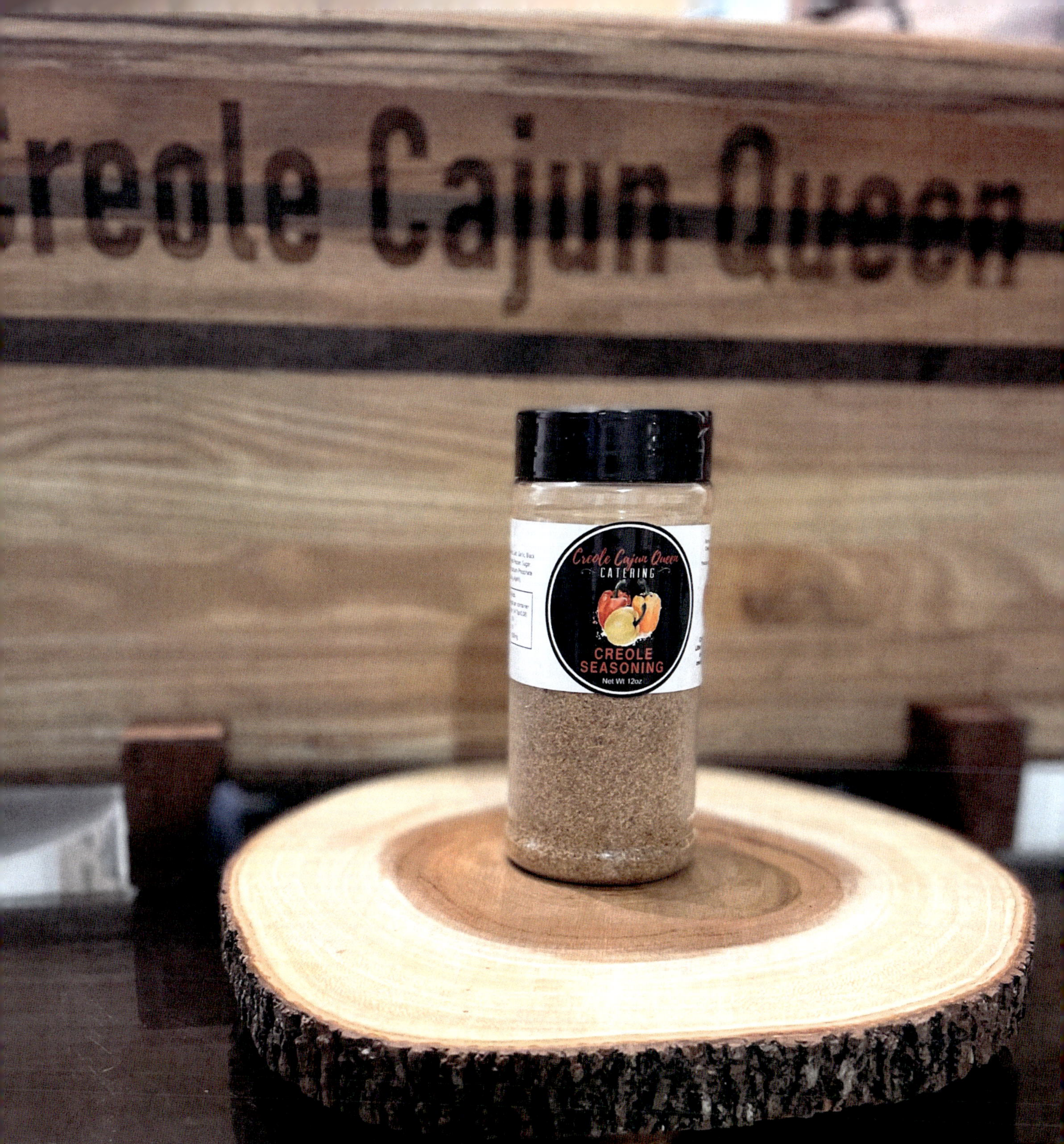
Cajun Queen
Creole Cajun Queen
CATERING
CREOLE
SEASONING
Net Wt 12oz

Creole Cajun Queen Smothered Cabbage

On the avenue is where I have great memories of this dish. Orleans avenue is where some of my siblings and I would meet up on some weekends play dominoes and watch my dad take out his big pot , chop up heads of cabbage, onions and salt meat to cook. My dad always talked himself through his cooking (lol). The conversation was just as good as the cooking.

The elements of good cooking begins with being able to explain why you use certain ingredients as much as using them. My dad was an inspirational cook. He was inspired by the tradition, the culture and the love of preparing foods that made your stomach smile. I could listen to him all day. And at the end of the day we would have good eating and even more GREAT conversation.

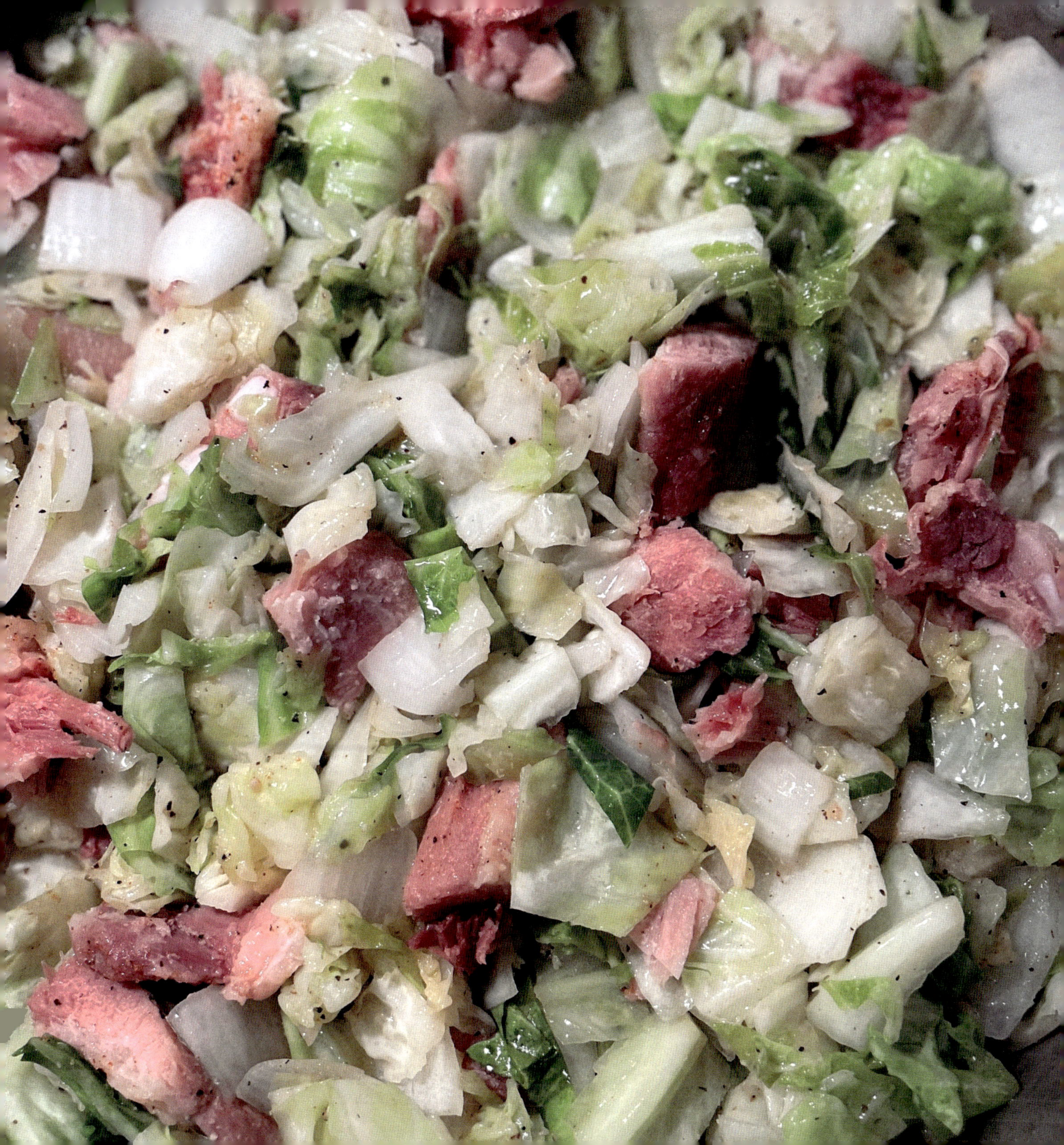

Ingredients

Serves 4-6

Serves 4-6
2 large Cabbage Heads
2 large onions
1 lb. pickled pork salt meat (smoke Turkey optional)
1/2 teaspoon salt
1/2 teaspoon black pepper
1 teaspoon Creole Cajun Queen Creole seasoning *(use any creole seasoning or order mine on line)*
1 teaspoon white sugar
1 tablespoon garlic powder
2 -3 tablespoon bacon grease

Instructions

1. Separate your dark cabbage and light cabbage greens. Wash and roll your darkest green cabbage first then cut into slices. Cut onions into 4 quarters.

2. Remove the stem off your cabbage head, cut the head down into 4 quarters and slice long ways then turn cutting your cabbage short ways

3. Boil your salt meat in a separate pot for 1 1/2 hour until tender. Drain water and set your meat aside.

4. In a large metal pot fry down your dark cabbage first with onions ,salt ,pepper , garlic powder, creole seasoning in your bacon grease. Cover your pot and allow your cabbage and onions to smother down on a low to medium heat for 15 minutes and then add your light cabbage for 20 more minutes.

5. Uncover your pot, add in your salt pork meat, sugar and stir until completely blended. Smother down for 15 minutes and serve.

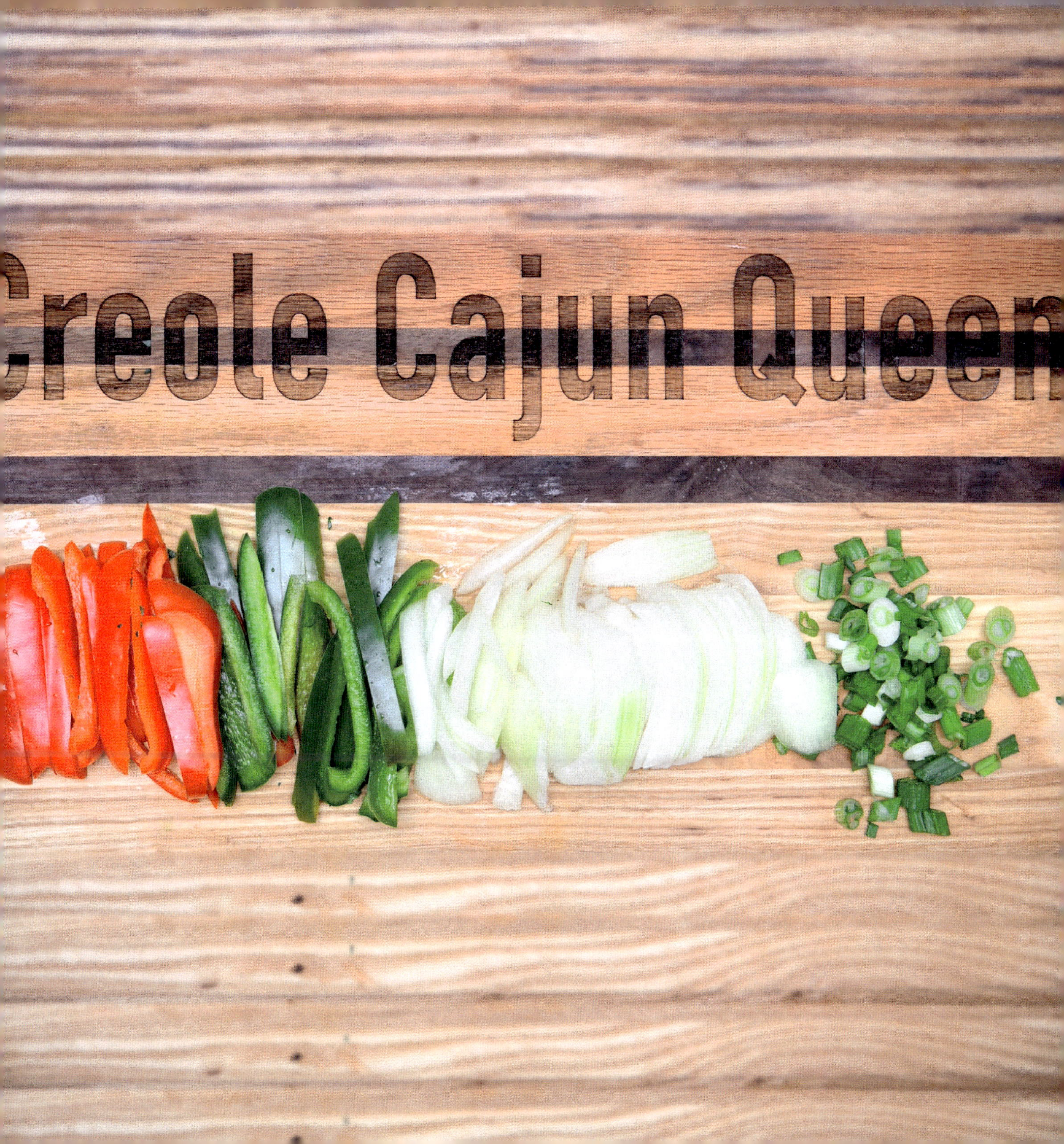
Creole Cajun Queen

Baaby Mac & Cheese Indeed

Mac and cheese is a special favorite for me. I call it hood Mac and cheese lol and that's because of the block cheese we use. I sat at a lot of tables in the 7th ward and studied a lot of the old schoolers on this recipe and then started adding different ingredients in my own way to get that creamy result. All of these ladies would say the same thing as I leave their kitchen... make sure your Mac and cheese is real cheesy.

Now let's be real here. Not everybody can make Mac and Cheese. Sure you can buy the box and heat it up, but what do you have really? A bowl of yellow stuff. The perfect Mac-N-Cheese requires skill, knowledge and a special something something that only comes from years of diligence, apprenticeship and have good eating and even more GREAT conversation.

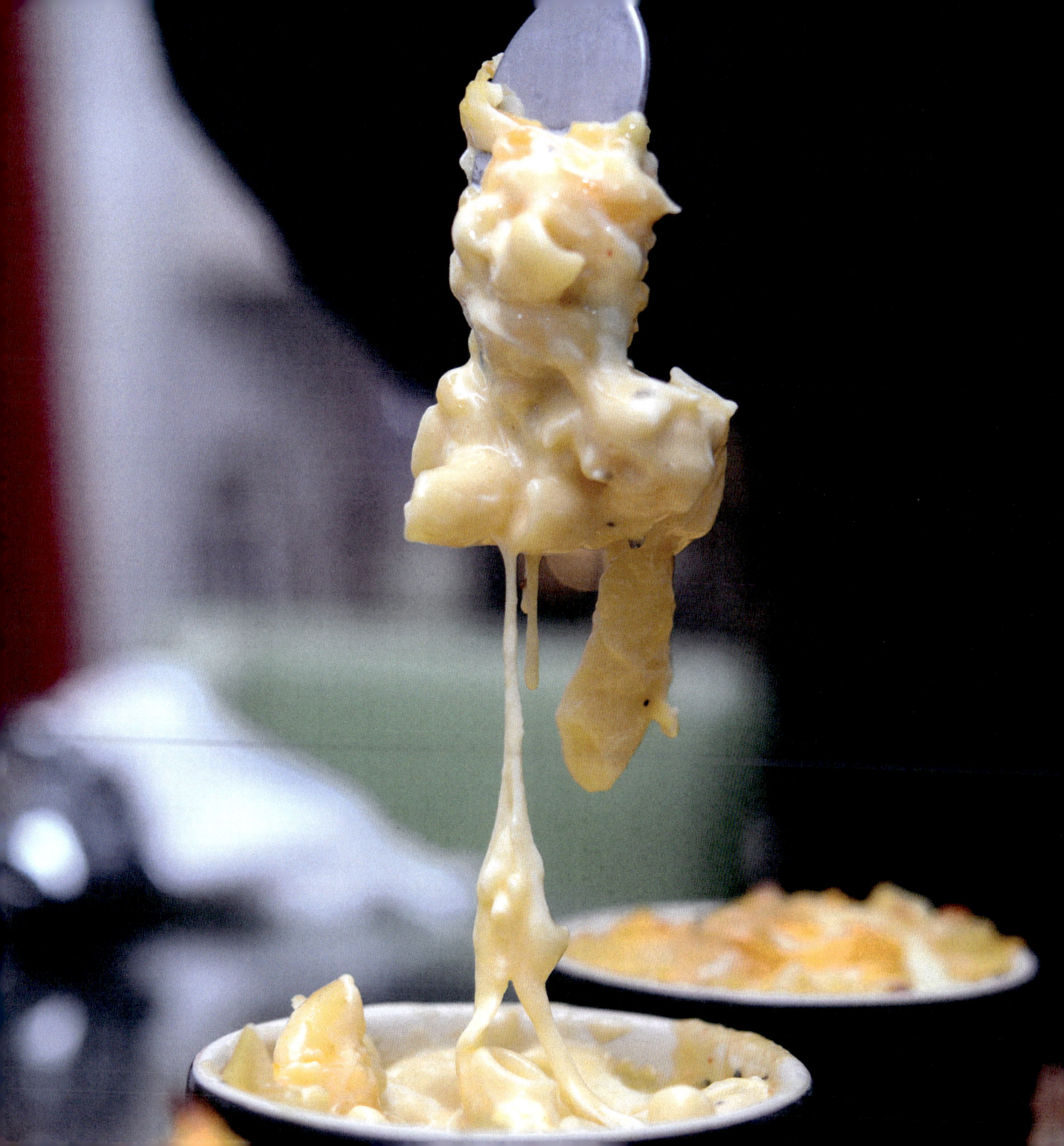

Ingredients

Serves 4-6

1 block American cheese
1 stick salted butter
2 cans cream
1 can cheddar cheese soup
1 can chicken broth
1 cup mozzarella Shred
1 cup Colby Shred
1/2 teaspoon salt
1 teaspoon black pepper
1 teaspoon white sugar
1lb large Elbow Pasta

Instructions

1. In a large pot bring water and 1/4 teaspoon salt to a boil for the pasta.
Boil until pasta is al dente (tender but firm), drain and wash in cold water. Set pasta in a baking dish aside.

2. In a sauce pan melt your block cheese, cheddar cheese soup, stick butter, cream and chicken broth whisking until creamy and smooth.

Set sauce aside

3. Salt and pepper your pasta.
Mix in 1/2 cup each of your mozzarella and Colby shred cheese.

4. Pour cheese sauce throughout entire pasta dish mixing it together until the pasta is fully covered.

5. Sprinkle the remainder of both shredded cheese until the pasta is covered, bake at 350 until the top cheese is melted and serve.

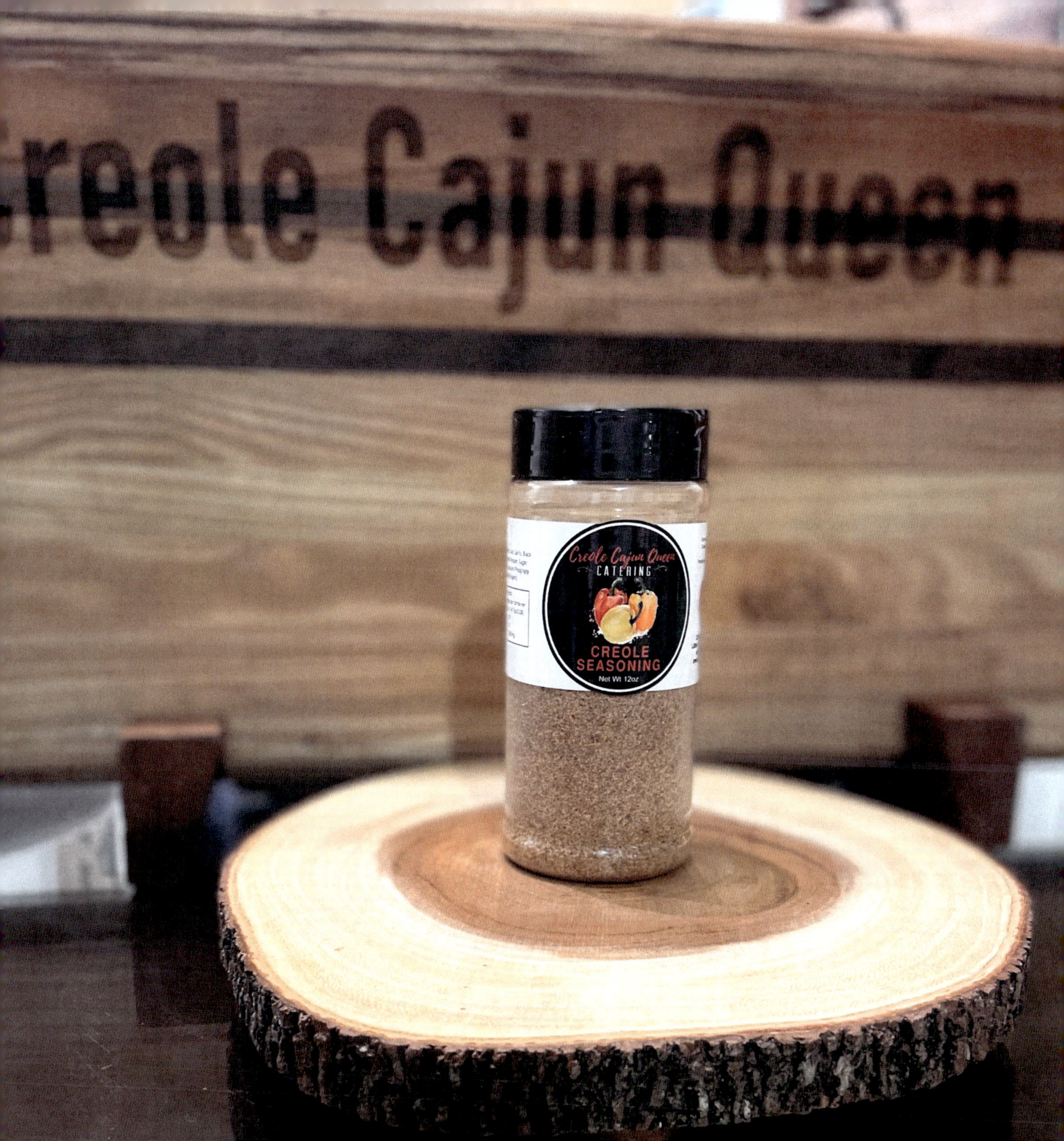
Creole Cajun Queen
Creole Cajun Queen
Catering
CREOLE
SEASONING
Net Wt 12oz

Creole Cajun Queen Shrimp and Grits

What can I say about shrimp and grits? Everything!!! If you're at a neighborhood seafood boil and you have left over shrimp... well in the morning shrimp and grits! A wedding, baby shower, brunch you name it!

At home shrimp and grits is a regular on many tables. Brown roux or cheese sauce your choice, shrimp and grits are the talk of the town.

Just writing about this dish puts me in a happy place.

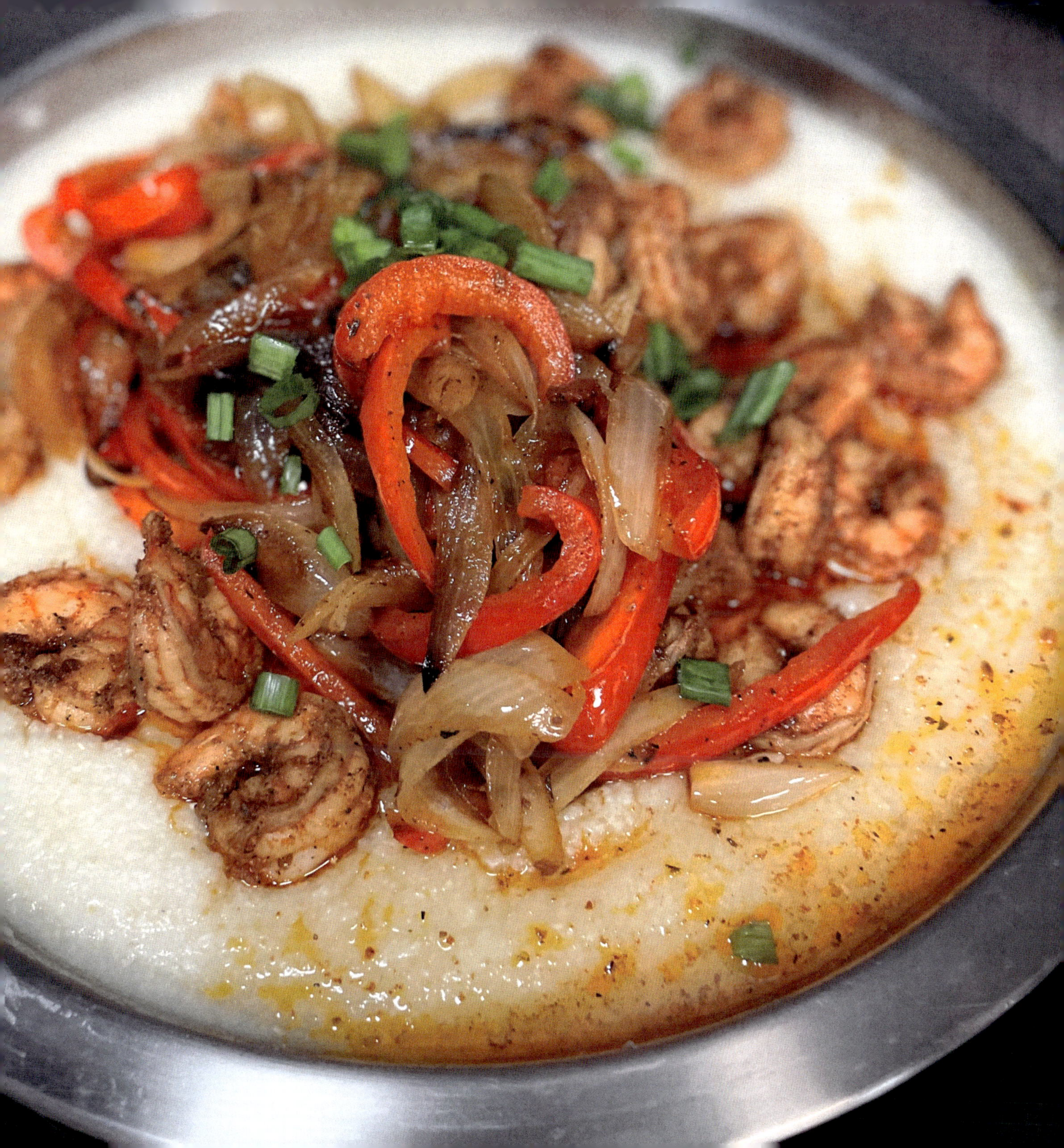

Ingredients

Serves 4-6

2 cups old fashioned cooked Grits (follow box instructions)
1 lb. peeled, deveined clean large Shrimp
1 yellow onion
1 red bell pepper
1/2 block American cheese
1 cup cheddar cheese
1 stick butter
1/4 teaspoon creole Cajun Queen creole seasoning *(use any creole seasoning or order mine on line)*
1/2 salt
1 pinch of cayenne pepper
1 tablespoon garlic powder
1 tablespoon black garlic
1 can of cream
1/2 can chicken broth

Instructions

1. Low to medium heat cook your grits. I follow the box directions but cook a little longer to make them super creamy. Add 1/2 stick of butter and salt to taste.

2. Season your shrimp, onions and bell pepper with black garlic powder. Sauté in a little butter until the shrimp is pink and seasoning is soft

3. Let's make the sauce. use your 1/2 block cheese,1/2 cup of cheddar cheese, 1 can cream, 1/2can chicken broth in a meal sauce pan blend together on a low heat stirring sauce until it becomes creamy. Add the garlic powder, cayenne pepper, creole seasoning, stir in evenly, turn your heat off and cover

4. In a bowl add your then your shrimp, onions and bell peppers. Next ladle your cheese sauce on top of your shrimp and grits. Eat and enjoy!

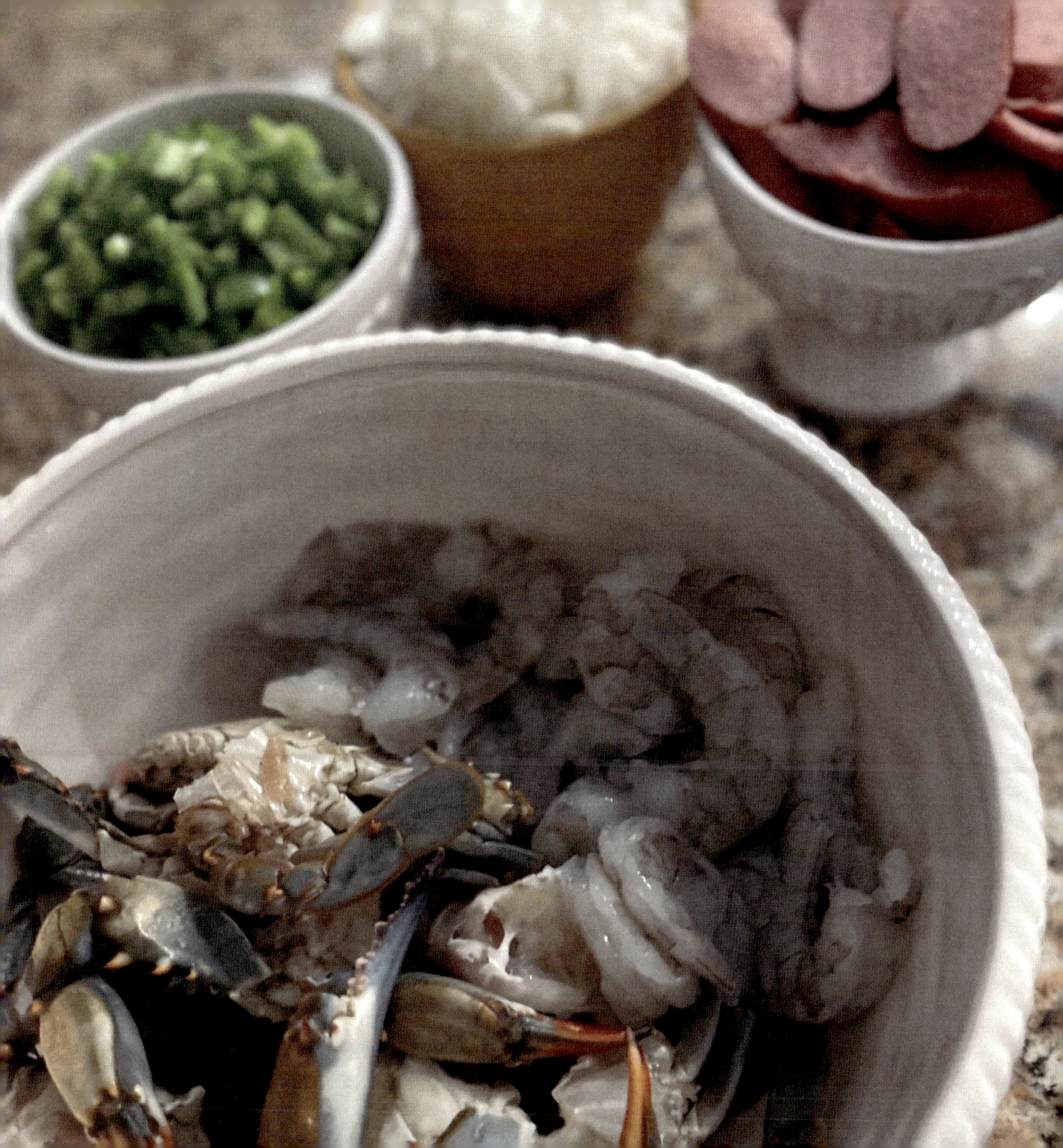

Back A' Town
Good Ole Fried Chicken

Good old fried chicken, at every corner store, gas station and of course at home, you name it! This southern comfort is even made as part of breakfast. I remember my Brother Curtis bringing me to New Roads, Louisiana as a kid and waking me up to Fried Chicken, Hot Creamy Grits, Biscuits and you name it. The Fried Chicken was always a memory connection for me when it comes to my brother and I, because he worked as a manager for Popeyes. It was walking distance from my elementary school and after school I remember having the delicious kids meals from there. Those memories still live inside of me.

But let make it perfectly clear. Just because you put grease in the skillet and drop chicken, don't mean you can fry "Good Ole Fried Chicken" There is a skill and an art to frying Good Ole Fried Chicken. First off it starts with seasoning and rubbing. (You have to rub the season in to get that get that Great "To the Bone" taste.)

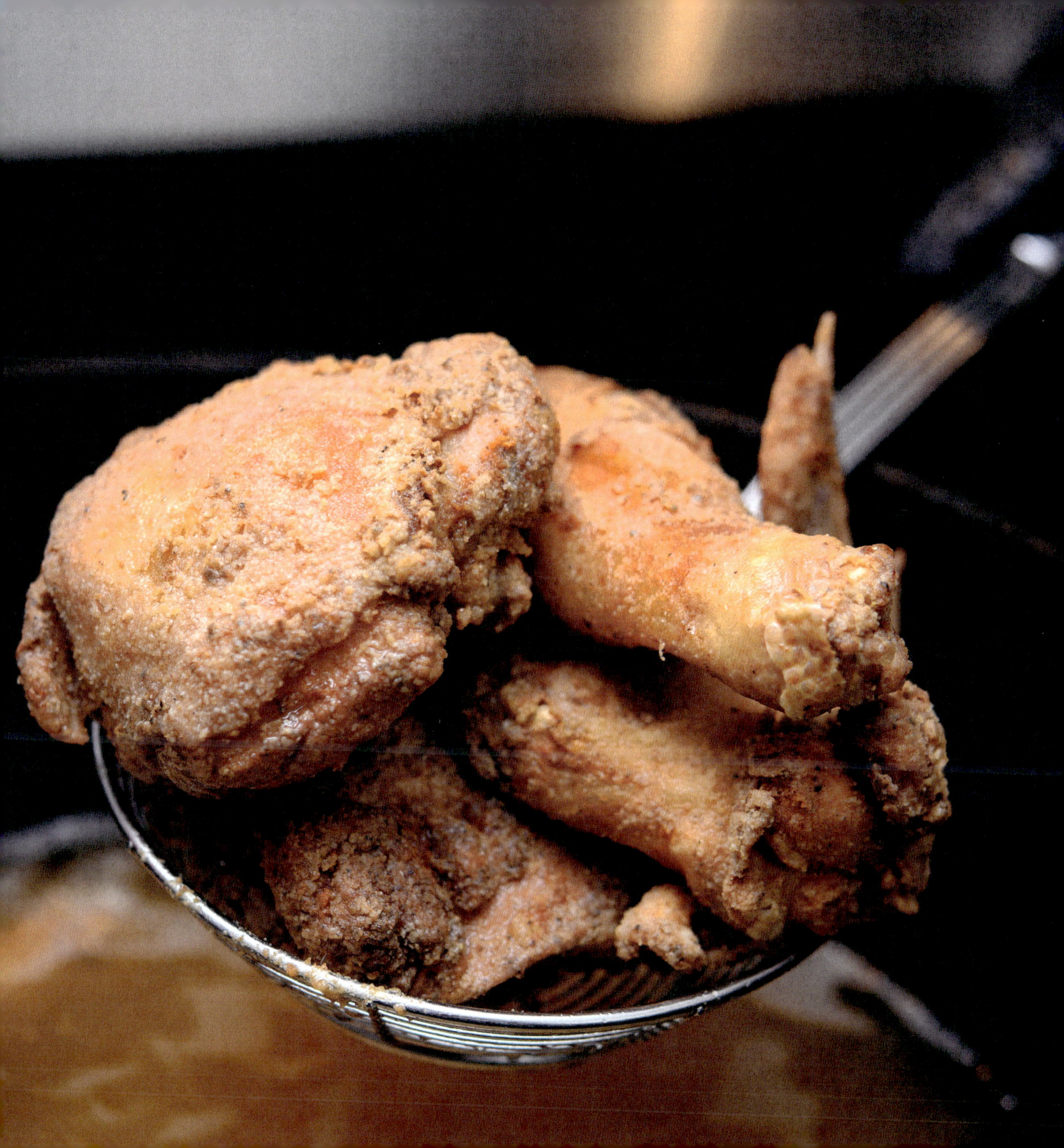

Ingredients

Serves 4-6

1 whole chicken
2 tablespoon Mustard
1 tablespoon garlic powder
tablespoon onion powder
1 tablespoon black pepper
1 teaspoon salt
1 teaspoon cayenne pepper
1 tablespoon creole Cajun Queen creole seasoning *(use any creole seasoning or order mine on line)*
3-4 cups Shortening (oil)
3 -4 cups of flour
1 brown paper bag

Instructions

1. Clean and cut up your chicken (already cut chicken is optional) pat dry and rub your mustard all over each part until fully covered. Season chicken with your dry seasonings, cover and chill in fridge for 2 hours or overnight if frying the next day.

2. Using a deep fryer or deep cast iron pot add your oil and heat to a 350 temp. Place your flour in the brown paper bag for shaking / coating your chicken. Sprinkle Creole seasoning in your flour.

3. Once your oil is hot, start adding your chicken a little at a time into your flour and shake until fully coated. Lay your chicken in oil. Fry until chicken floats and temp at 365. Drain your chicken on a paper towel plate and eat.

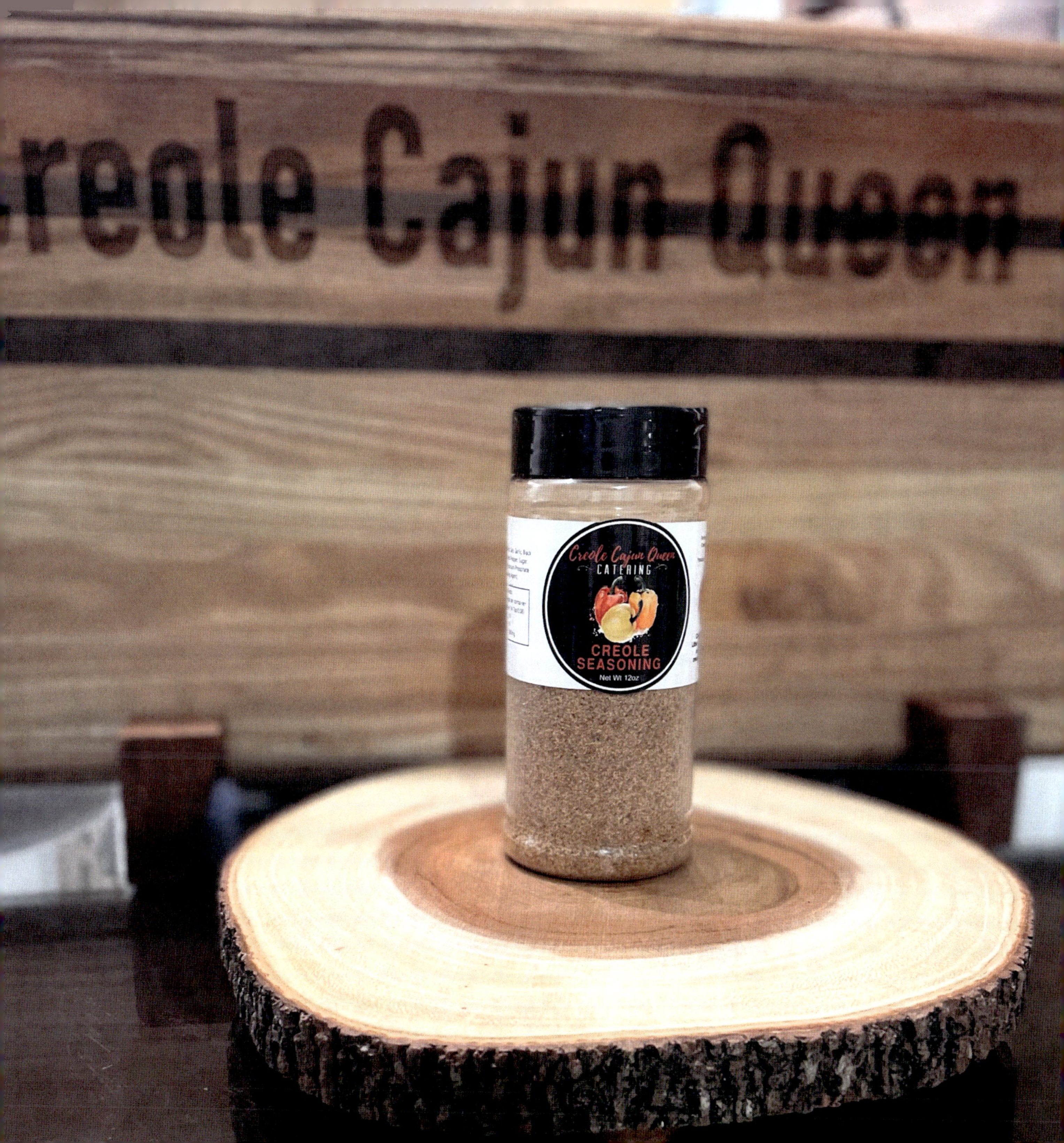
reole Cajun Queen
Creole Cajun Queen
CATERING
CREOLE
SEASONING
Net Wt 12oz

Creole Cajun Queen Crab Cakes

Crab cakes was my "eat lite before I go out" food. Crab cakes was served on many brunch buffets in the hotels in New Orleans. For many of my younger years I worked as a waitress at the famous Baileys restaurant inside the Fairmont hotel. This place taught me that Crabcakes can be served with any meal.

I learned at this hotel that I would be tied to creating dishes forever. I served Mayors, governors and celebrities. I watched the head chef make these awesome cakes and perfected them with my own touch rub the season in to get that get that Great "To the Bone" taste.

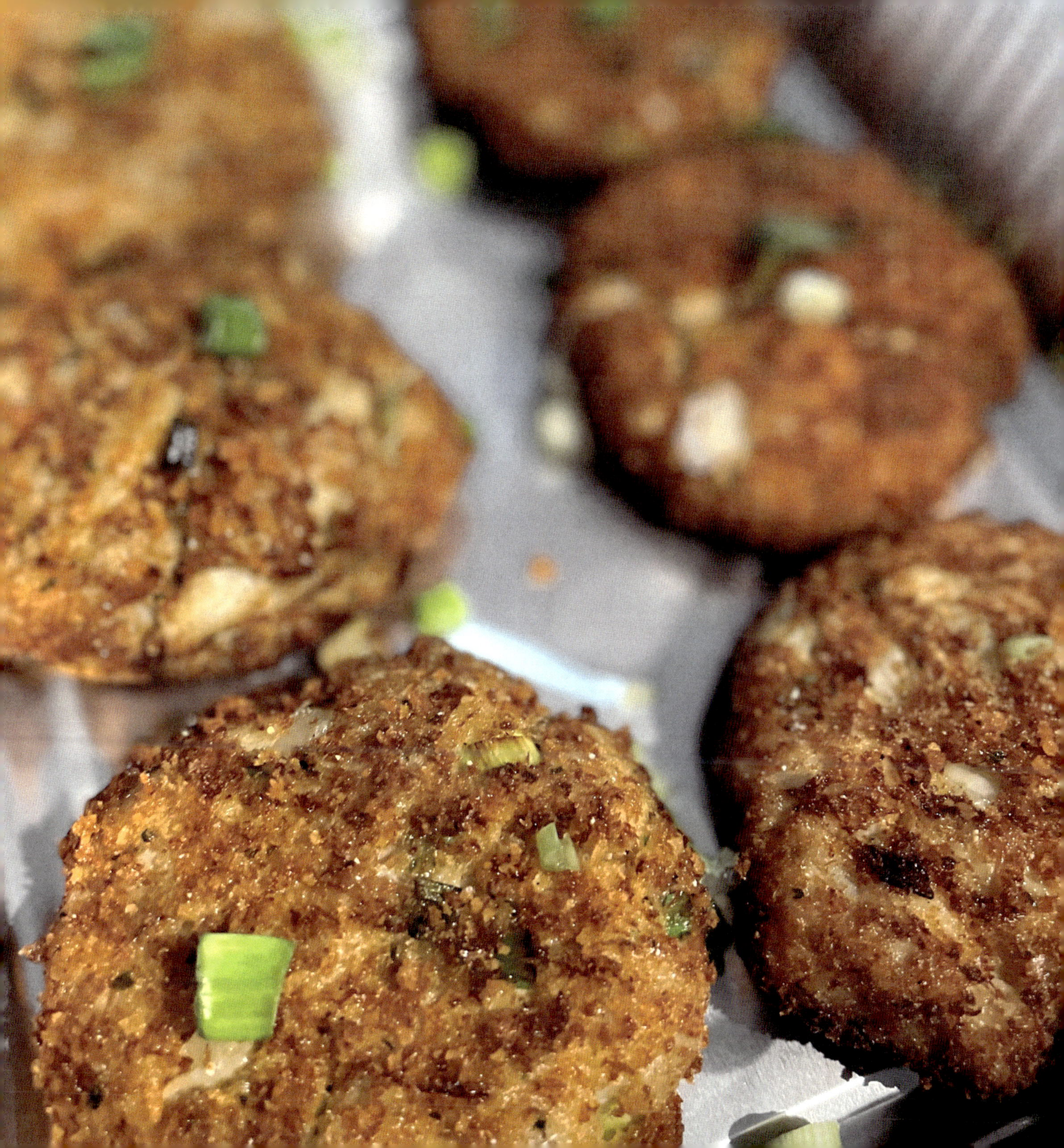

Ingredients

Serves 4

16 ounces Lump Crab Meat
3 eggs
1 tablespoon green onion
1 teaspoon white onion
1 1/2 tablespoon blue plate mayonnaise
1 teaspoon creole mustard
1/2 teaspoon garlic powder
1/4 teaspoon black pepper
1 pinch cayenne pepper (optional)
1/2 teaspoon chop Italian parsley
1/4 teaspoon Creole Cajun Queen creole seasoning *(use any creole seasoning or order mine on line)*
1 cup bread Italian crumbs
3 cups cooking oil

Instructions

1. Empty your crab meat in a bowl. Dice /chop your white onion, green onion and parsley then add into the crab meat.

2. Sprinkle in your garlic powder, 2 tablespoon bread crumbs, black pepper, cayenne pepper, creole seasoning, 1 egg, mustard and Mayo, then mix all together.

3. Set up your station using a bowl with 2 eggs and 1 tablespoon water mixed for dipping and a bowl with bread crumbs to coat your crab cake. Pour 3 cups of oil in a deep metal fry pan. Heat to 350.

4. Once the crab is mixed start scooping your mix into the palm of your hand rolling it in a ball (an ice cream scoop is fine), dip first in egg wash then roll in bread crumbs evenly. Form until it starts sticking together. Slightly flatten and keep the round shape.

5. Fry on each side 2-3 minutes or until light golden brown. Drain on a paper towel, plate and serve.

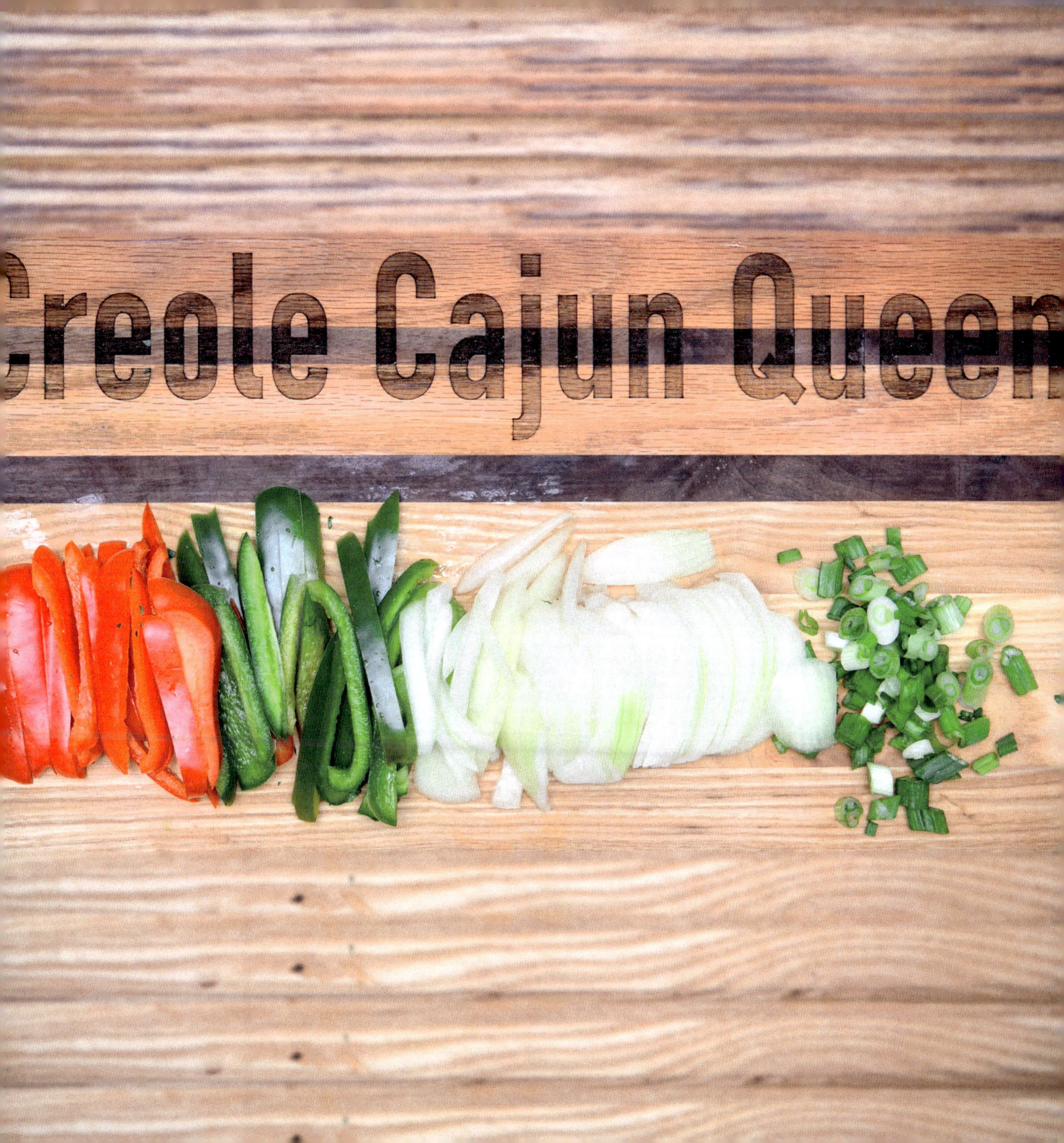
Creole Cajun Queen

Creole Cajun Queen Crab & Shrimp Corn Bisque

Cooking this bisque gave me so much peace. I have tasted several around New Orleans but this was one of my recipe challenges when I became divorced. The time it took to get the ingredients together and cook floated me into another place. I would grab me a glass of wine, put on my music and play around with getting my flavor just right. My sister would just rave about this dish lol

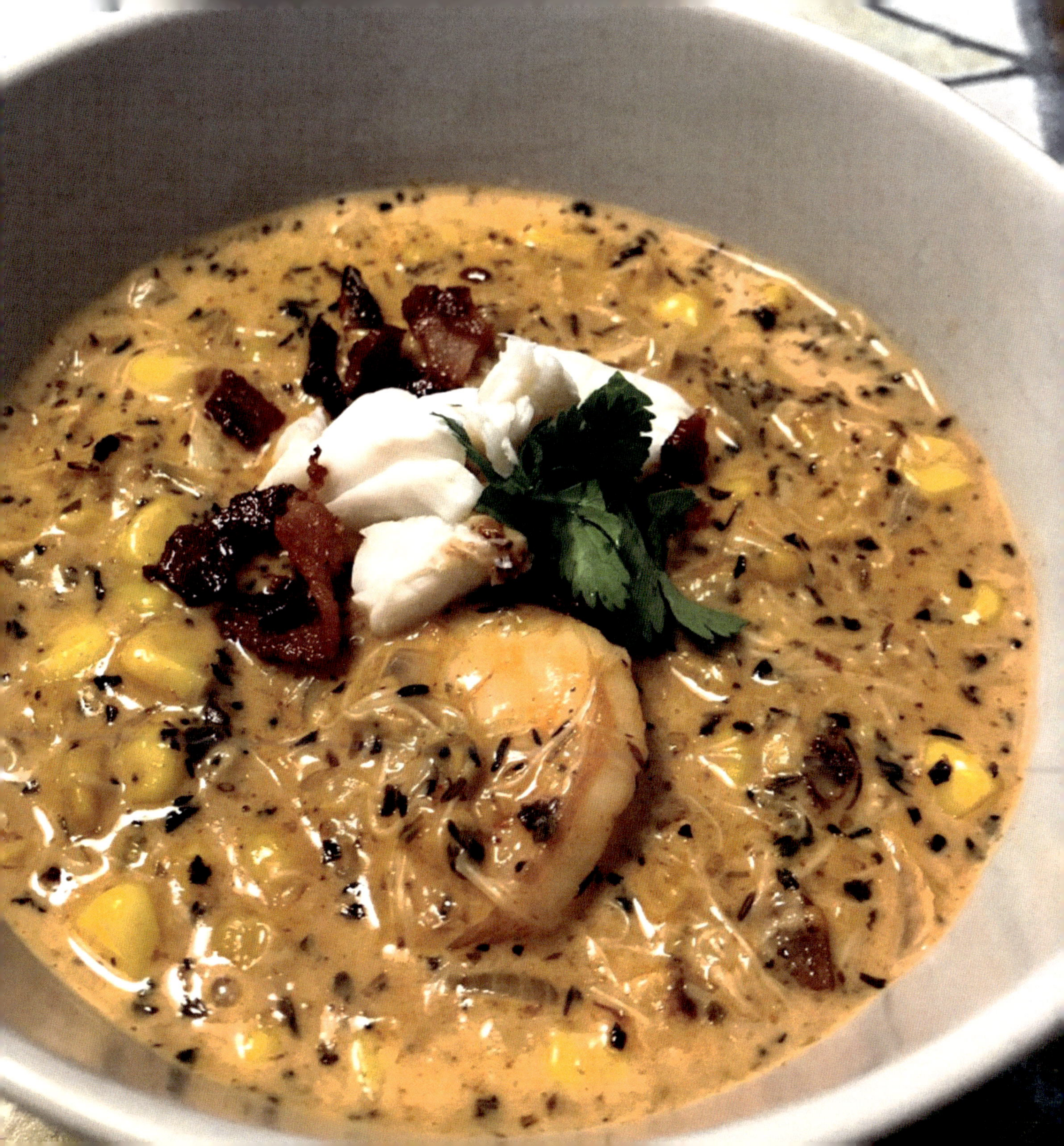

Ingredients

Serves 4-6

6 ears of fresh cob corn
1 stick margarine
1 stick butter
1 bunch green onions
1 lb. lump crab meat
1/2 pound thick Bacon
1 lb. peeled, cleaned deveined
1 can cream corn
1 teaspoon kitchen bouquet
1 8oz cream cheese
1 can of chicken stock
1 cup shrimp stock
1 yellow onion
1 red bell pepper
1 tablespoon creole Cajun Queen creole seasoning *(use any creole seasoning or order mine on line)*
1 teaspoon crab boil (powder form)
1 tablespoon garlic powder
1 teaspoon thyme
1 teaspoon crush garlic
1 cup cheddar cheese
1 bunch fresh Italian parsley
Use salt to taste

Instructions

1. Dice up your onions, bell pepper, and green onion. Shuck your corn and using a butter knife shave the corn kernels off of the cob into a bowl. Dice and cook your bacon.

(continued on next page)

Instructions (continued)

2. In a metal or cast iron skillet melt your margarine and butter. Sauté the fresh corn, bacon, onions and bell peppers until soft.

3. Sauté your shrimp, crab meat and green onions together with your corn.

4. Add in your chicken stock, shrimp stock, cream corn, and cream cheese stirring together on a low to medium heat.

5. Once the bisque began a small boil, Lower heat and add gradually the cheddar cheese, kitchen bouquet, garlic powder, crab boil, creole seasoning, crush garlic and thyme whisking/simmering together.

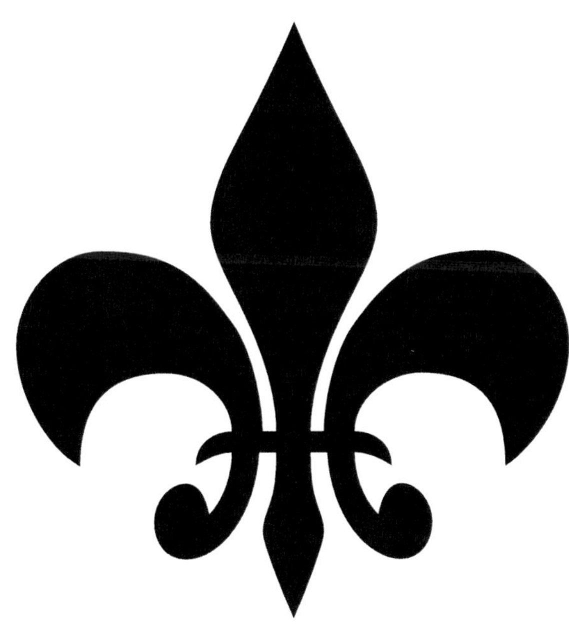

Creole Cajun Queen Slow Cooked Pot Roast

Pot Roast is one of my funniest disaster cooking stories. I had to practice and practice this Sunday favorite. I remember trying to impress a boyfriend and cook a pot roast, gravy, rice, green peas and oh yes potato salad. I must have put enough grease to fry chicken to make my roux for my roast lol. I pan seared the roast so black I had to scrape with a butter knife to get the burnt pieces off Lawd!!! I called my cousin for help and she laughed so much until I just hung up, Anyway you get the picture with that roast. When done right it can be AMAZING. When done wrong it can be AWFUL.

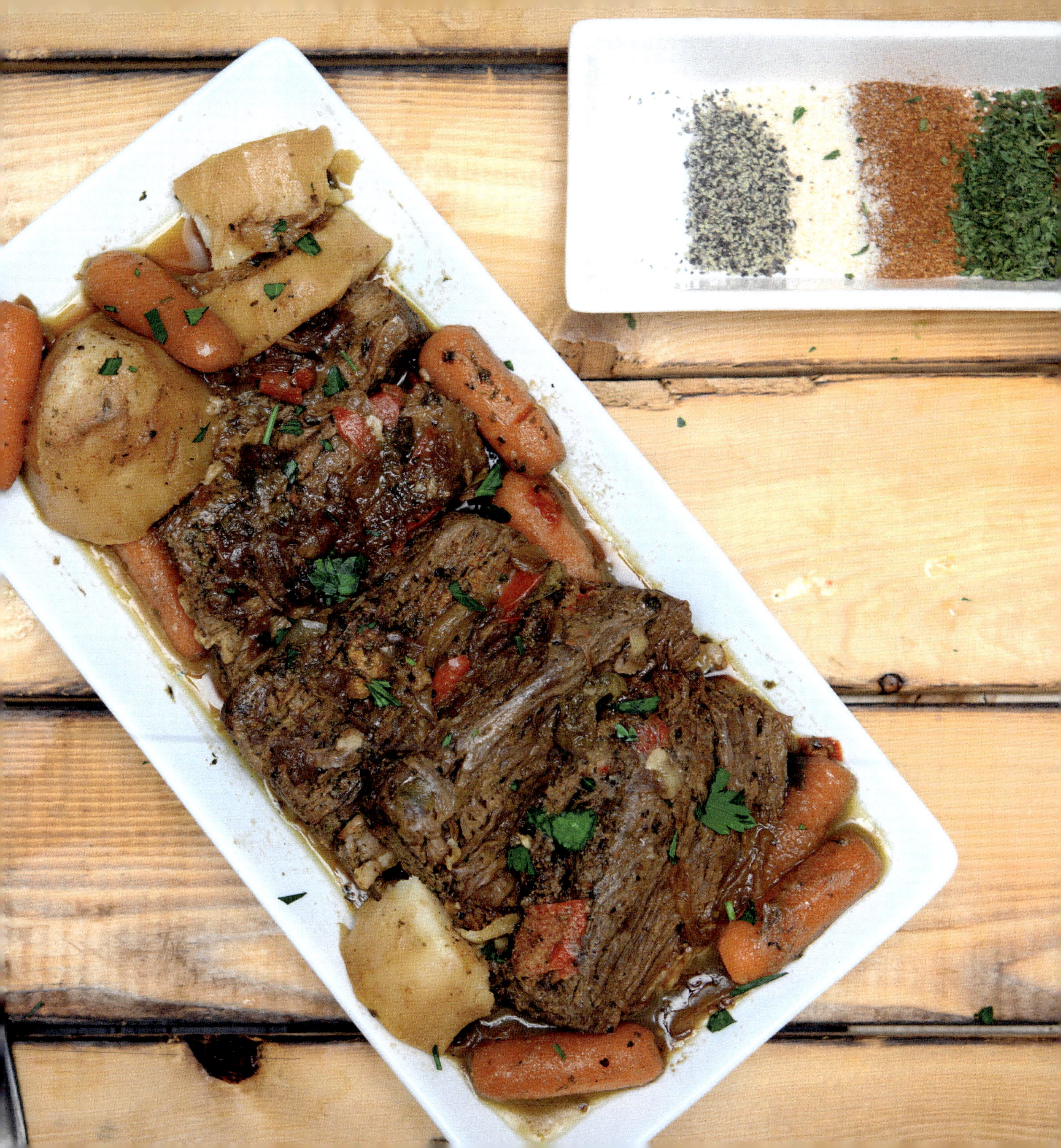

Ingredients

Serves 4-6

1 chuck Roast
1 yellow onion
1 green bell pepper
1 bunch green onion bulb (remove grassy strings in the end)
1 garlic bulb peeled
1 tablespoon Creole Cajun Queen creole seasoning *(use any creole seasoning or order mine on line)*
1/2 teaspoon salt
1 teaspoon black pepper
1 teaspoon garlic powder
1 tablespoon fresh Italian parsley
2 cups cooked rice
3 tablespoon vegetable oil
1 stick salted butter
1 cup white flour

Injection sauce:

1 cup water
1 tablespoon garlic powder
1/2 teaspoon accent
1/2 teaspoon creole Cajun Queen creole seasoning *(use any creole seasoning or order mine on line)*
2 tablespoon Worcestershire sauce . Whisk together blending evenly. This should not be pasty add water to loosen.

Instructions on Next Page

Instructions

1. Wash, clean and dry your roast. Make tiny slits and stuff with your fresh garlic and green onion bulbs. Slice your onions and bell peppers.

2. Start injecting your roast with the injection mix all over in the metal pot you are cooking/ finishing it in. Season your roast with salt, pepper and garlic powder. Cover and Refrigerate overnight.

3. Remove from fridge add in 3 tablespoon oil to the bottom of the pot. Heat on top stove on a medium heat. Allow the roast to lightly fry turning on each side. Once fried lightly remove from roast and set aside in a bowl.

4. In the same pot add in another tablespoon of oil let it get hot and 1 cup flour. Keep stirring until the flour mix is a pecan brown. The roux will become pasty but keep stirring on a low heat. Once the color is there and your kitchen is filled with this awesome aroma and smoke lol, toss in 1/2 onions and 1/2 bell peppers slices, mix it in with your roux.

5. Add in 1 can of beef stock, 1 cup water. Blend your roux mix in with your liquids evenly then Add your roast back to the pot top with remaining onions and bell peppers. I make sure my liquids slightly cover my roast add more stock or water if needed. Drop more of your dry seasonings to the pot stir then top with your Italian parsley cover and run it in your oven on 350 for 3 hours. Serve over rice and enjoy!

Creole Cajun Queen Red Beans and Rice

Red Beans and rice is a Monday tradition in my neighborhood. The school cafeteria even served red beans and rice on Mondays. This dish have the locals in love, but for the families in my neighborhood it was a stretch meal for the lower income. I would drive across the I-10 and at the very top between canal exit and the Elysian Fields exit you can smell the aroma from different people homes cooking their red Beans. I mean literally you can roll your windows down and smell it in the air. My Mom taught me you must soak your beans the night before and to start off with less water than the package calls for or they will not come out creamy.

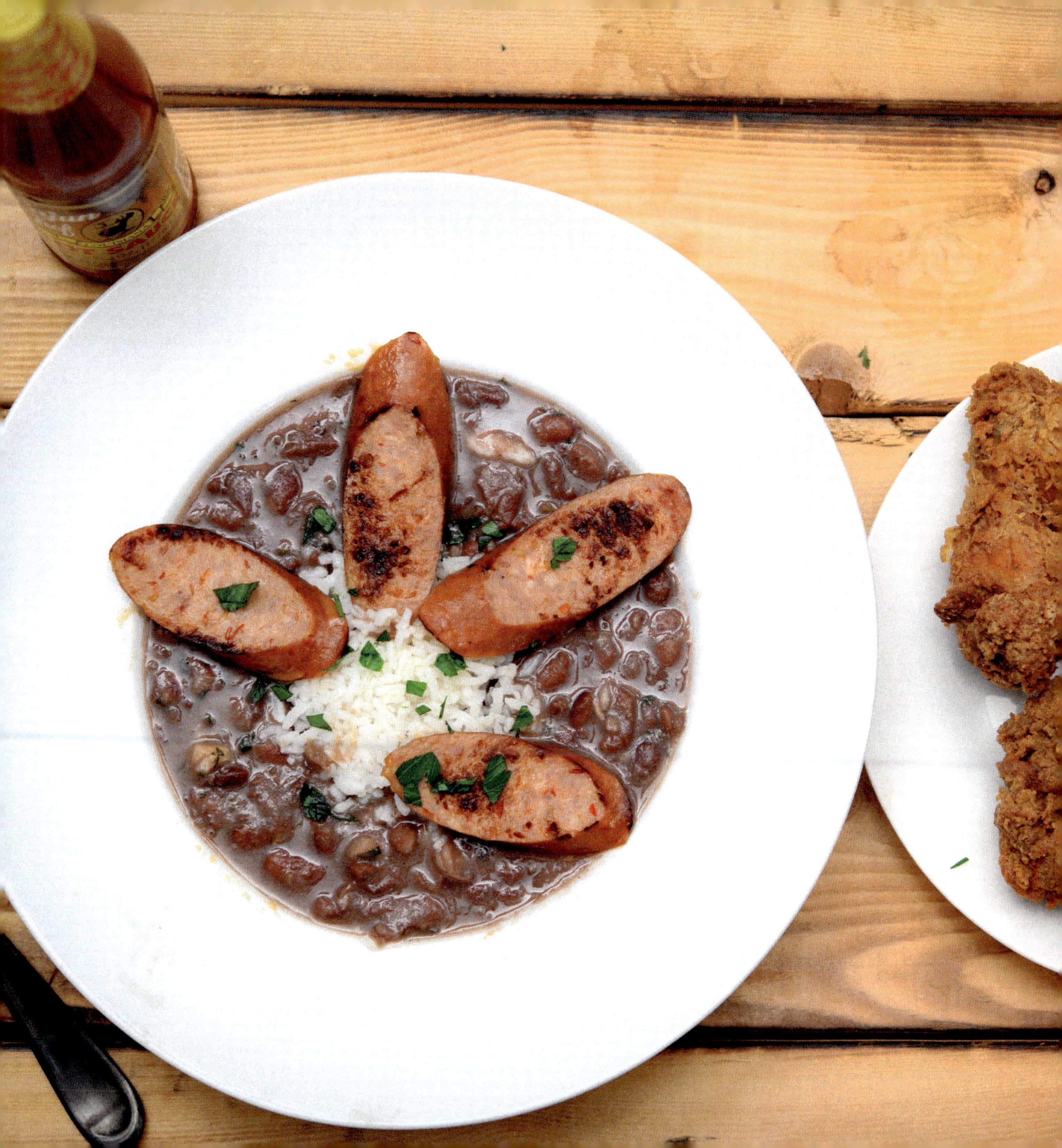

Ingredients

Serves 4-6

1 Pack dry Camellia Red Kidneys beans (pre-soaked covered with water overnight in the fridge)
1 yellow onion
1 green bell pepper
1 lb. smoke sausage
1 lb. pickled meat (ham seasoning option)
1 tablespoon creole Cajun Queen creole seasoning *(use any creole seasoning or order mine on line)*
1 teaspoon salt
1 teaspoon black pepper
1 tablespoon garlic powder
1 tablespoon onion powder
A pinch of white sugar
1 cup Italian parsley
3-5 cups water
2 cups cooked white rice

Instructions

1. Pull your pre-soaked beans from the fridge. Rinse then in a cast iron or metal pot on a medium heat add 2 cups of water slightly covering your beans .Dice your bell peppers and onions and add to your pot. I like to start off cooking my beans with my diced seasoning.

2. In another pot boil your pickled meat for an hour. Boiling this meat helps to take some of the salt out. Set aside when done. If you are using ham seasoning I normally fry it down before adding it to the beans.

3. Bring your beans to a nice boil checking your water level for about 1-2 hours. Cover your pot and keep on a low to medium heat. Slice your sausage and add to your pot.

(continued on next page)

Instructions (continued)

4. While your beans are still cooking add in another cup of water and stir. The package calls for 5-6 cups of water but I don't add all at one time to monitor my beans becoming too watery

5. At the second hour your beans should have start to become soft and your bean juice a little thick. With your cooking spoon start smashing some of your beans against the sides of the pot, this helps them become creamier. Add in you pickled meat or ham seasoning and stir. Add in another cup of water, toss in your dry seasoning and parsley, stir while smashing a little more beans, cover and simmer for another hour on low- medium heat.

6. 3 hours in your beans should be soft, nice and creamy. Serve over a bed of rice, sprinkle with more parsley and serve.

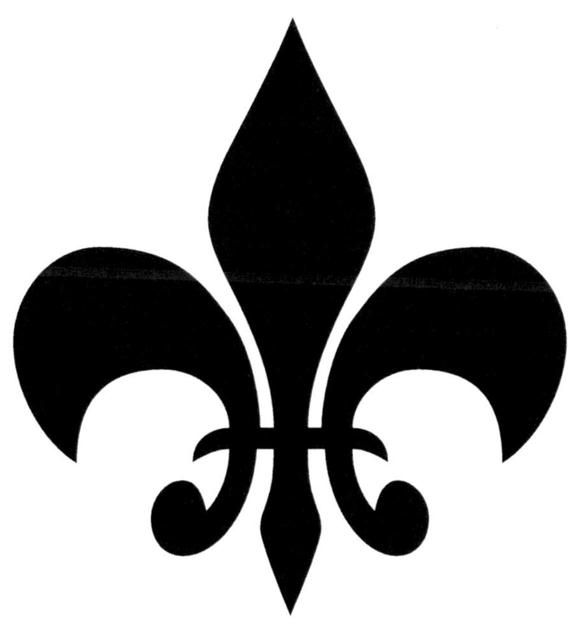

Creole Cajun Queen Shrimp Pasta

This pasta was my first hustle while working for the electric company. I worked in the credit and collection department and being a single mother selling supper plates as we called it was a good way to earn extra money. My job started at 8 am and I would get up at 5am make this pasta, package them in containers and sell to my co workers for lunch. This pasta helped me perfect my cooking skills .

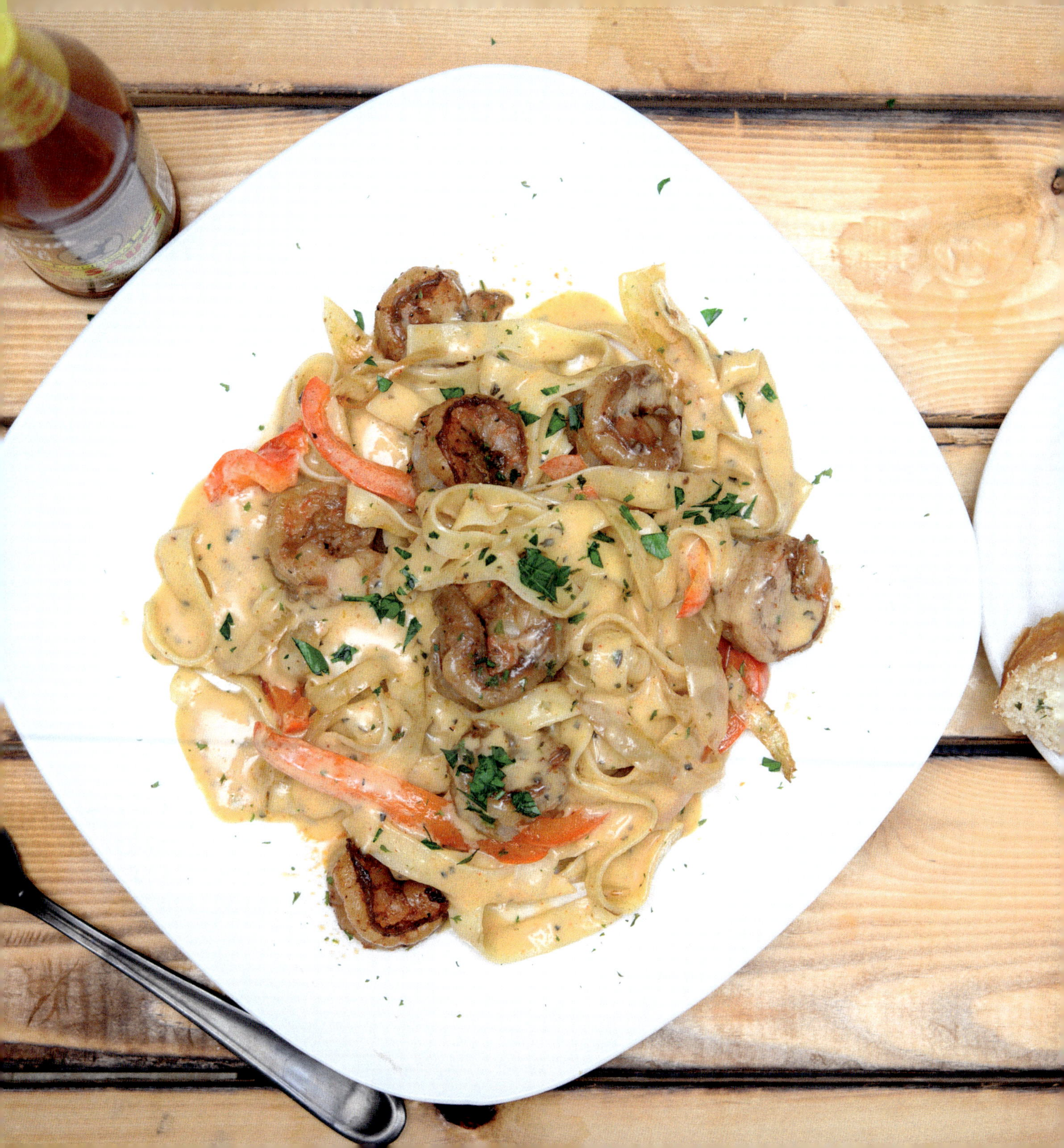

Ingredients

Serves 4-6

1 lb. peeled, clean, deveined large shrimp
1 -16oz pack wide fettuccine pasta
1 red bell pepper
1 green bell pepper
1 yellow onion
1 cup green onion
2 cloves fresh dice garlic
1 tablespoon fresh Italian parsley
1 teaspoon creole Cajun Queen creole seasoning *(use any creole seasoning or order mine on line)*
1 stick margarine
1 teaspoon basil
1 tablespoon garlic powder
1/4 teaspoon crab boil (powder form)
1/4 teaspoon black garlic
1 teaspoon smoked paprika
1 teaspoon white sugar
2 cans cream
1 block American cheese
1 can cheddar cheese soup
1/2 can Chicken broth

Instructions

1. In a deep pot, boil your pasta until tender but firm (al dente). Sprinkle a little salt in your water at the beginning of your boil. Rinse pasta with cold water oil with olive oil and season your pasta with the black garlic and basil, (I preseason all my pastas baby!)Evenly mix. Set aside.

(continued on next page)

Instructions (continued)

2. Season your shrimp, bell peppers, onions with black garlic powder and smoked paprika. Pan Fry your shrimp in a small frying pan 3 minutes on each side, medium to high heat until the shrimp has a blackened look and sauté bell peppers, onions dice garlic set aside.

Sauce:

4. In a metal sauce pan add your cream, chicken broth, block cheese and 1 stick of margarine whisking over a low to medium heat until smooth and melted. Add in your shrimp, bell peppers, onions and garlic

5. Add in your basil, crab boil, creole seasoning, and garlic powder and stir blending in with your sauce.

6. Pour sauce over your pasta mix add in your green onions, plate, then top with chopped Italian parsley and serve.

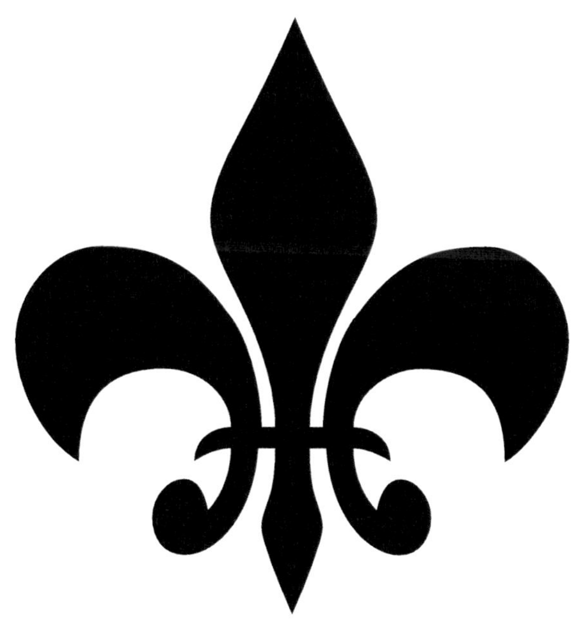

Dirty, Dirty DIRTY Rice

Dirty rice is my OMG! Recipe because even some people in New Orleans says “I don’t eat dirty rice with chicken livers” and that’s why I eat Popeye’s dirty rice lol ha ha, well you do!

Authentic dirty rice is made with chicken livers with no meat. I add meat because I like the way the pork sausage makes my flavors pop! But however you make “real Dirty Rice” it will make the meal turn out right. Often when folks are craving Cajun Creole Cusine, they ask for Dirty Rice. Rice is such a staple that anyway it’s prepared is amazing. I call this my OMG Recipe because that’s the response I get every time I make it. It’s not uncommon to hear someone say…

”You put your FOOT in that there”

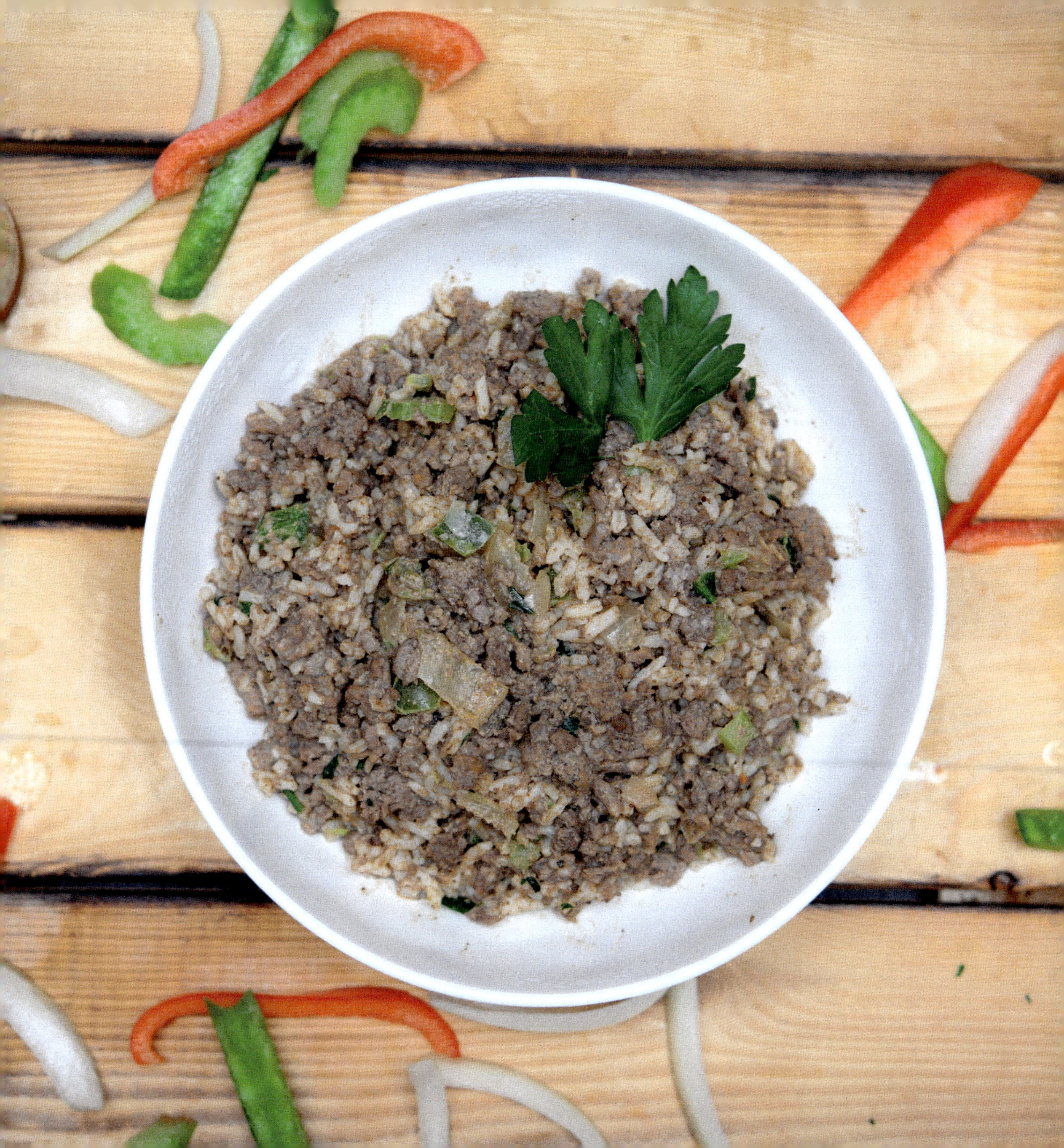

Ingredients

Serves 4-6

2 lb. long grain cooked white rice
1/2 container chicken livers
1/2 lb. spicy pork sausage
1 yellow onion
1 green bell pepper
1 red bell pepper
2 long celery sticks
1 cup green onion
1 /2 teaspoon salt
1 teaspoon black pepper
1 tablespoon garlic powder
1 pinch of cayenne pepper
1 teaspoon Creole Cajun Queen creole seasoning *(use any creole seasoning or order mine on line)*
1 /2 cup chopped Italian parsley
1/2 stick margarine
1 tablespoon cooking oil (your choice)
2 tablespoon white flour
2 tablespoon water
1 cap full liquid crab boil

Instructions

1. First I boil my chicken livers in a little bit of water and crab boil. A 30 minute boil is fine and set aside. Next I cook my pork sausage until all the pink is gone. You will need a blender or food chopper to blend up your chicken livers. I blend it up to a liquid. This plays a big part in your dirty rice sauce mix. Set aside.

(continued on next page)

Instructions (continued)

2. In my cast iron pot (Juanita is my favorite cast iron) I heat it up on a medium to high heat fire and add both my margarine and oil. Once my pot is hot I add in my onions, celery, bell peppers and garlic stirring together until they are soft.

3. Next I add my flour stirring it in my seasoning mix. I make just a little bit of a roux so if you need just a tiny bit more of oil this would be fine. Stir until you see a little bit of a browning color watching your heat.

4. After you see a little bit of browning going on add in you chicken livers mix , pork sausage ,green onions, parsley and water and mix all together evenly.

5. Now that your mix is all blended start mixing in your cooked rice and your dry seasonings. Mix evenly. Your rice should look just like the name dirty rice. We serve it with anyone of our favorite meat on the side.

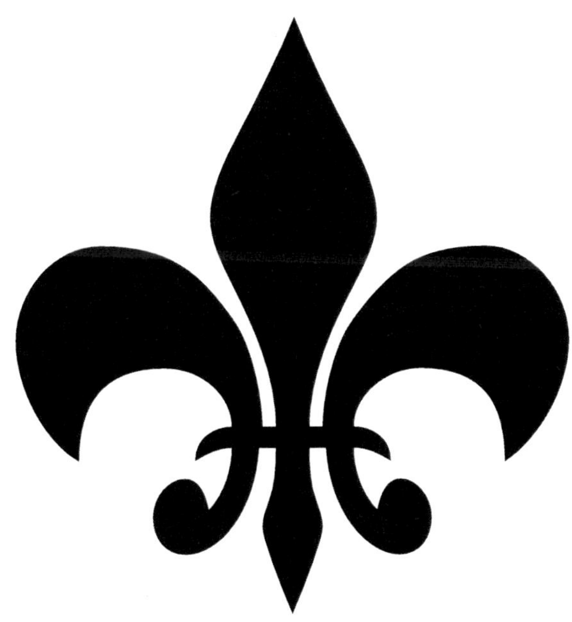

Creole Cajun Queen Stuffed Chicken Breast

My stuff chicken breast is an entertaining hit! When I started catering I would offer this dish. I truly believe all New Orleanians sit back and think of things to stuff lol. I hope this simple dish be the talk of your parties as it has been for mine. It's been said that you can't mess up chicken. I beg to differ. I have seen many times that chicken was too dry or rubbery.

This Stuffed Chicken Breast is a crowd pleaser and is often requested. By adding a crab meat and sausage stuffing, it takes a tried and true favorite and makes it a special entree that will be enjoyed again and again. If you are looking for that one dish that folks will all remember you for...THIS IS IT!!!

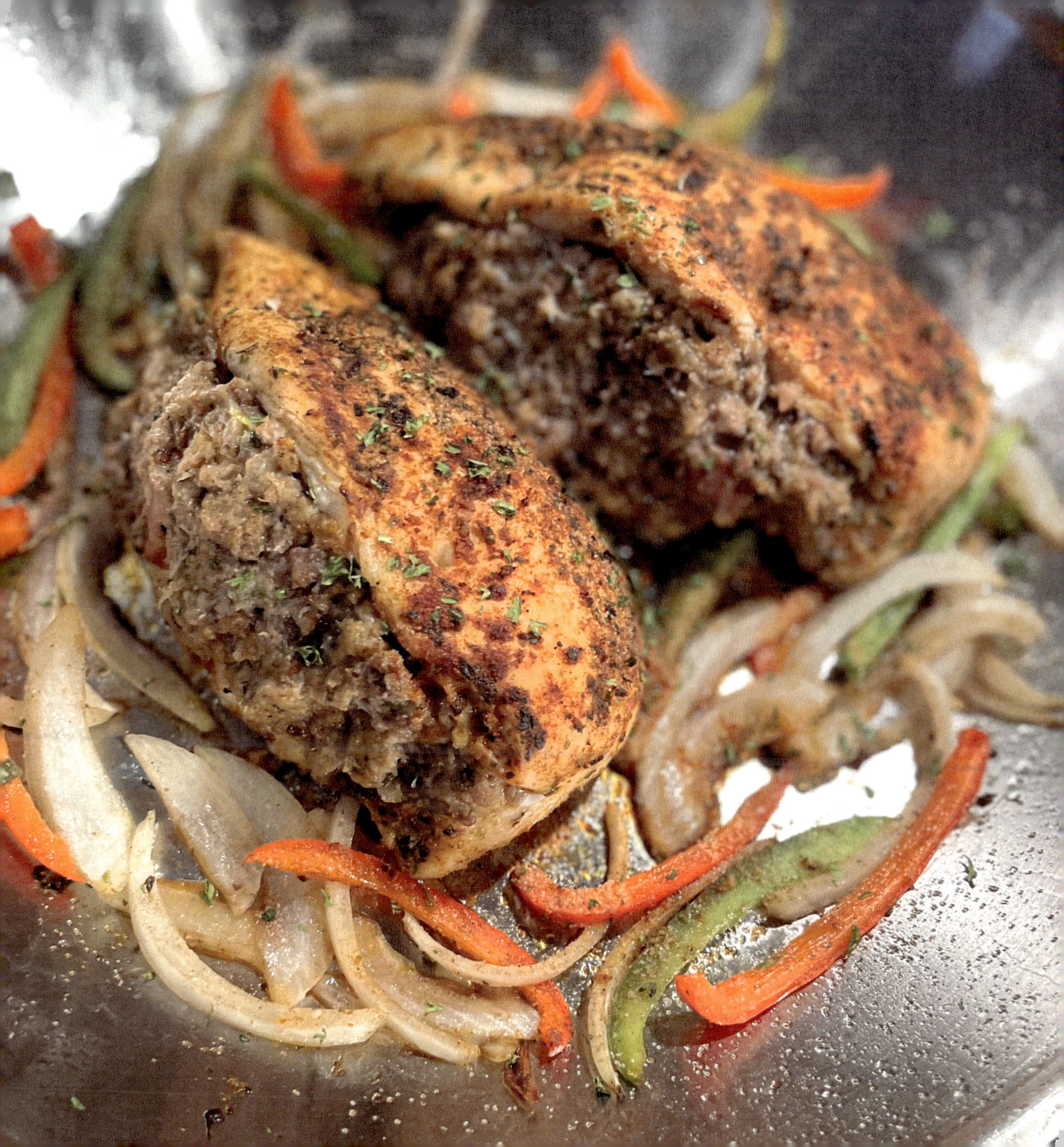

Ingredients

Serves 4

4 skinless thick chicken breast
1 lb. spicy Italian sausage
1 lb. lump crab meat
4 cloves of garlic
1 yellow onion
1 cup green onion
2 tablespoon fresh chopped Italian parsley
1 cup seasoned breadcrumbs
1 green bell pepper
1 red bell pepper
1 tablespoon garlic powder
1 teaspoon black pepper
1 teaspoon smoked paprika
1 tablespoon onion powder
1 teaspoon Creole Cajun Queen creole seasoning *(use any creole seasoning or order mine on line)*
1 8 oz. can chicken broth

Instructions

1. Take your cleaned chicken breast and make deep slits in the center of the meat. Dry your meat, oil it with olive oil and season with creole seasoning, garlic powder and smoked paprika. Dice up your onions, garlic, parsley and bell peppers. Set aside.

2. In a medium fry pan on medium heat, fry down your Italian sausage removing all pink, add in your onions, bell peppers and garlic in with your sausage and mix together.

(continued on next page)

Instructions (continued)

3. Once your meat mixture is cooked add in your lump crab meat. Give it a stir all together. Next add in Your dry seasonings and mix. cut your fire; add in your bread crumbs and chicken broth gradually. Mix together until it becomes like a moist stuffing. Mix in your fresh parsley last and set aside.

4. In another fry pan add in a tablespoon of olive oil, heat up to a medium to high heat. Once the oil is heated lightly fry your chicken breast on each side getting a nice blackened coating and remove to cool for stuffing.

5. Using a tablespoon start scooping your mix into the slits of your chicken breast and hold your chicken breast together with toothpicks. Bake in the oven on a greased baking dish at 350 for 20 minutes. I usually cover it with foil to keep the moisture of the meat. Cool for 5 to 10 minutes and enjoy!

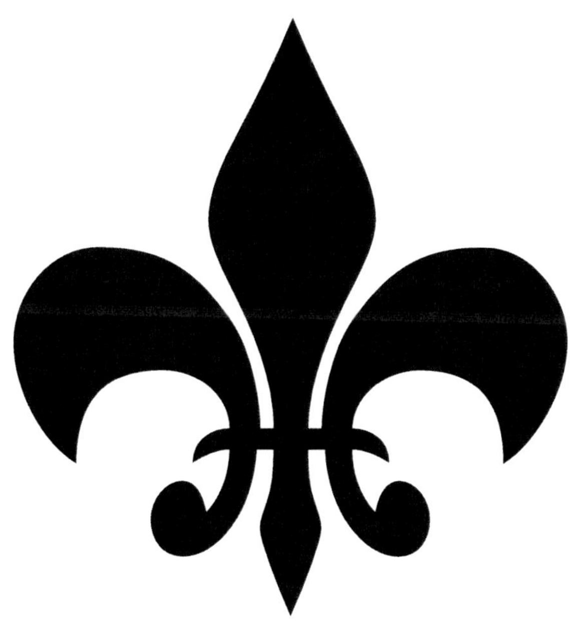

Garlic Butter Shrimp and Sausage Pasta Yvette

This recipe was inspired by one of the women who loved me like a daughter (Ms. Yvette) my daughter's grandmother. MS Yvette would cook for anyone who was at her home on Sunday mornings. She would start off with cooking breakfast and stole my heart with this dish. I took this dish added some of my own twist and made it my own.

This is one of my best signature pastas. There is just something special, and unique about a perfectly presented pasta. The shrimp in that buttery savory sauce is good enough by itself. When I add the sausage it adds a unique extra taste that makes your stomach smile. Every time I prepare this dish I am reminded of my daughter and her daddy's mother. It reminds me of what family and friendship is all about.

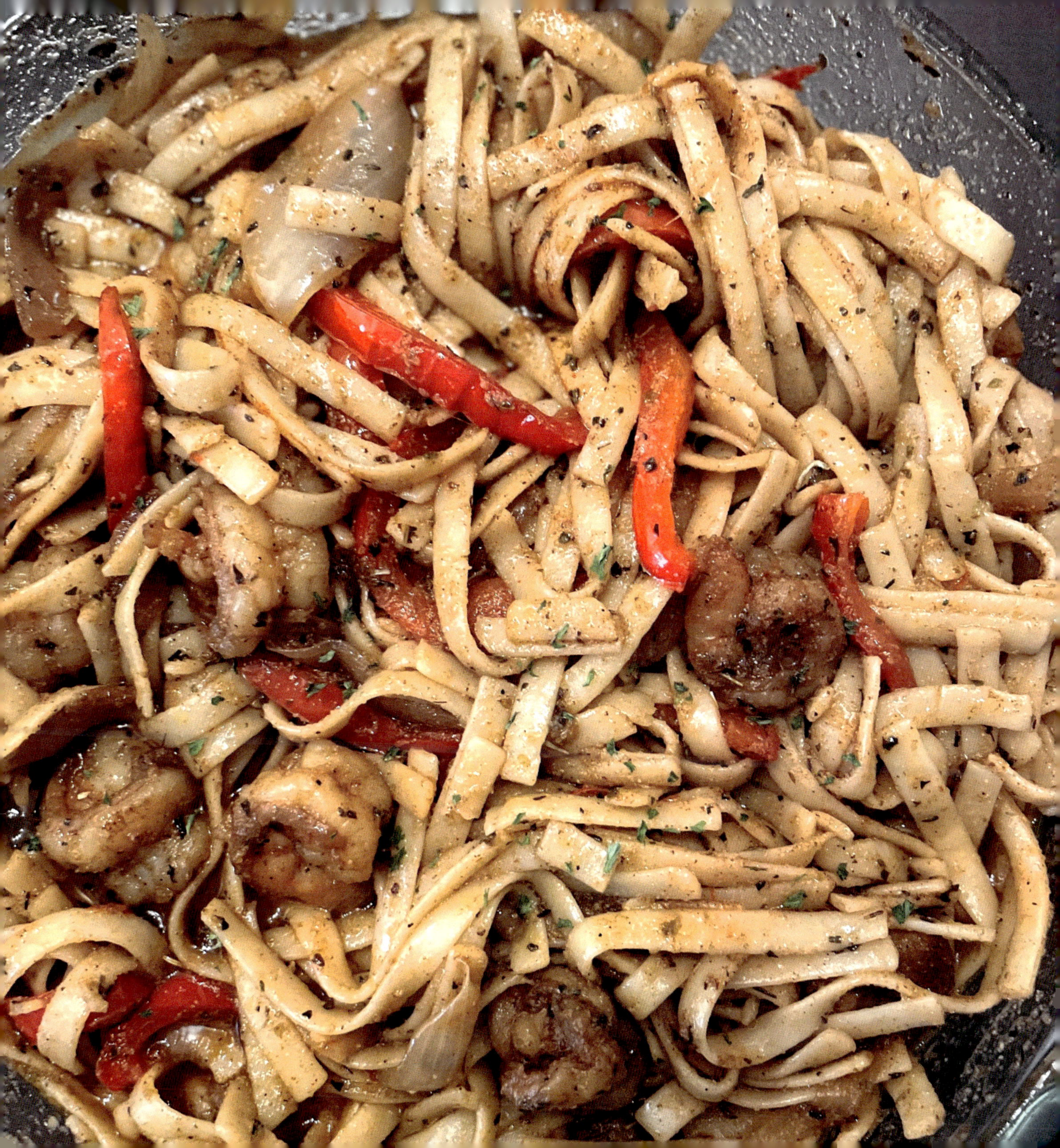

Ingredients

Serves 4-6

1 pack of cooked linguine or fettuccine
1 lb. peeled, clean and deveined shrimp
1 lb. smoke sausage
1 red bell pepper
1 green bell pepper
1 yellow onion
1 tablespoon Italian seasoning (dry)
1 teaspoon basil (dry)
1/2 teaspoon cayenne pepper
1 teaspoon Creole Cajun Queen creole seasoning *(use any creole seasoning or order mine on line)*
2 tablespoon garlic powder
1 tablespoon black garlic powder
1 teaspoon black pepper
2 sticks of margarine (if you want it really saucy add more margarine)
1 tablespoon soy sauce
A pinch of salt

Instructions

1. Slice up your onions, bell peppers (Jillian/ long ways) and smoke sausage (round sliced) season your shrimp with black garlic powder. Set these ingredients aside.

2. I use a heavy metal pot. Heat 1 stick of margarine on a medium fire. Once the pot is hot add in your bell peppers, onions and sausage. Fry down mixing together until the seasoning is soft but firm and sausage is browned. Set aside.

3. In the same pot fry in your shrimp until pink. Next toss back in your onions, bell peppers and sausage with more margarine, soy sauce and your dry seasonings. Once it's well mixed well cut your fire off and mix in your pasta. Your pasta is ready to serve and eat.

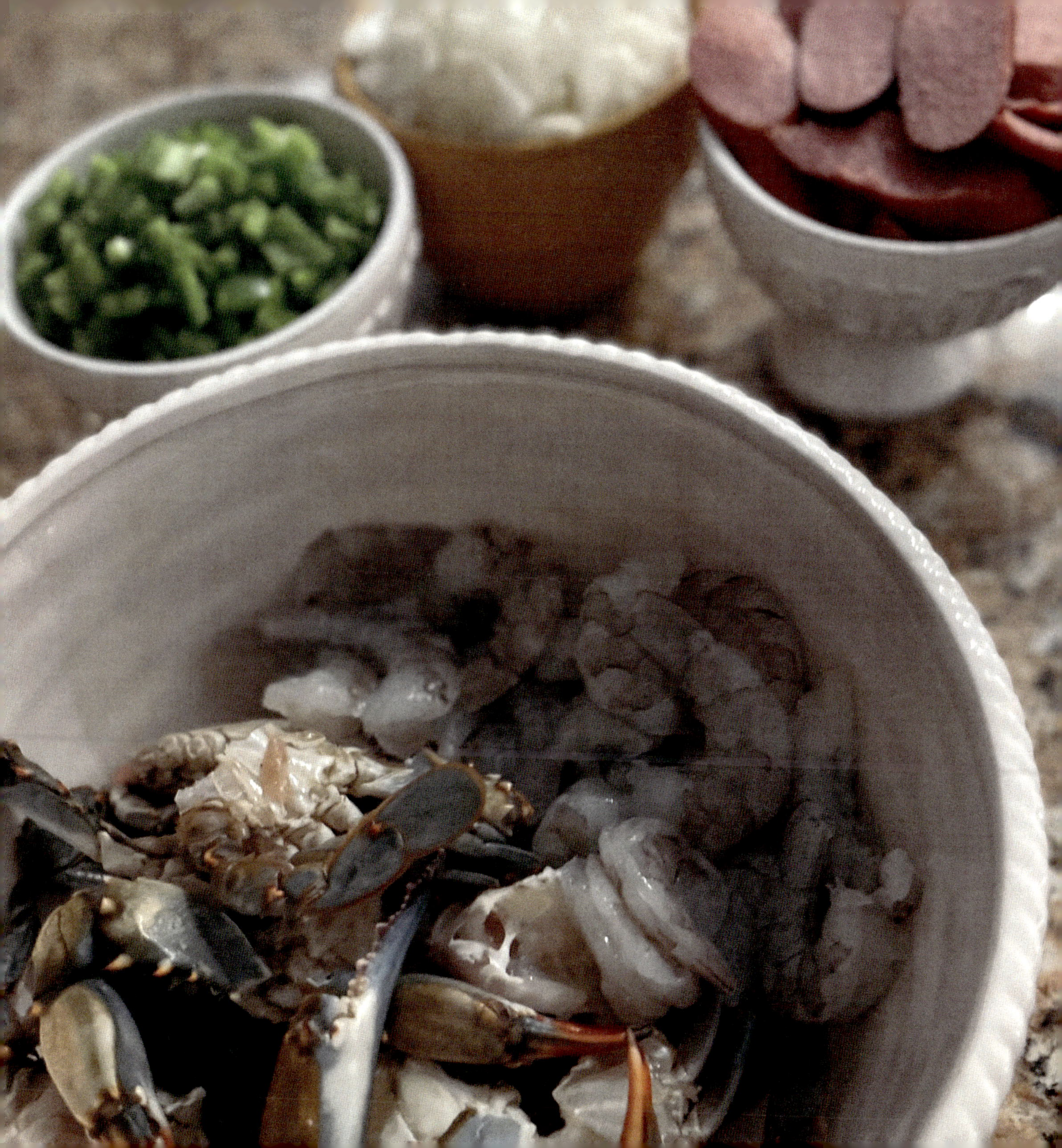

Oxtails, Smothered Nice and Slow

I have cooked oxtails twice in New Orleans but in Texas I am cooking this delicious meal often. I think about one of my favorite Chefs' (Julia Childs) when I am cooking this meal mainly because of the wine and butter lol.

Putting on my music and having a glass of wine watching this meal cook nice and slow keeps me in a relaxed moment. One thing for certain, Oxtails ain't cheap. When I go to the grocery to get the needed ingredients, sometimes I just have to shake my head. But then I realize that they are more than worth it. Ask anyone that had a pot of oxtails cooked nice and slow. Everyone will tell you that this is a meal that will warm up a cold night. Cooking them "Nice & Slow" makes them tender and delicious. You will see grown men sucking every last morsel of meat and savory goodness off of an oxtail. It is truly a work of art to see a pot of them being enjoyed by true oxtail lovers.

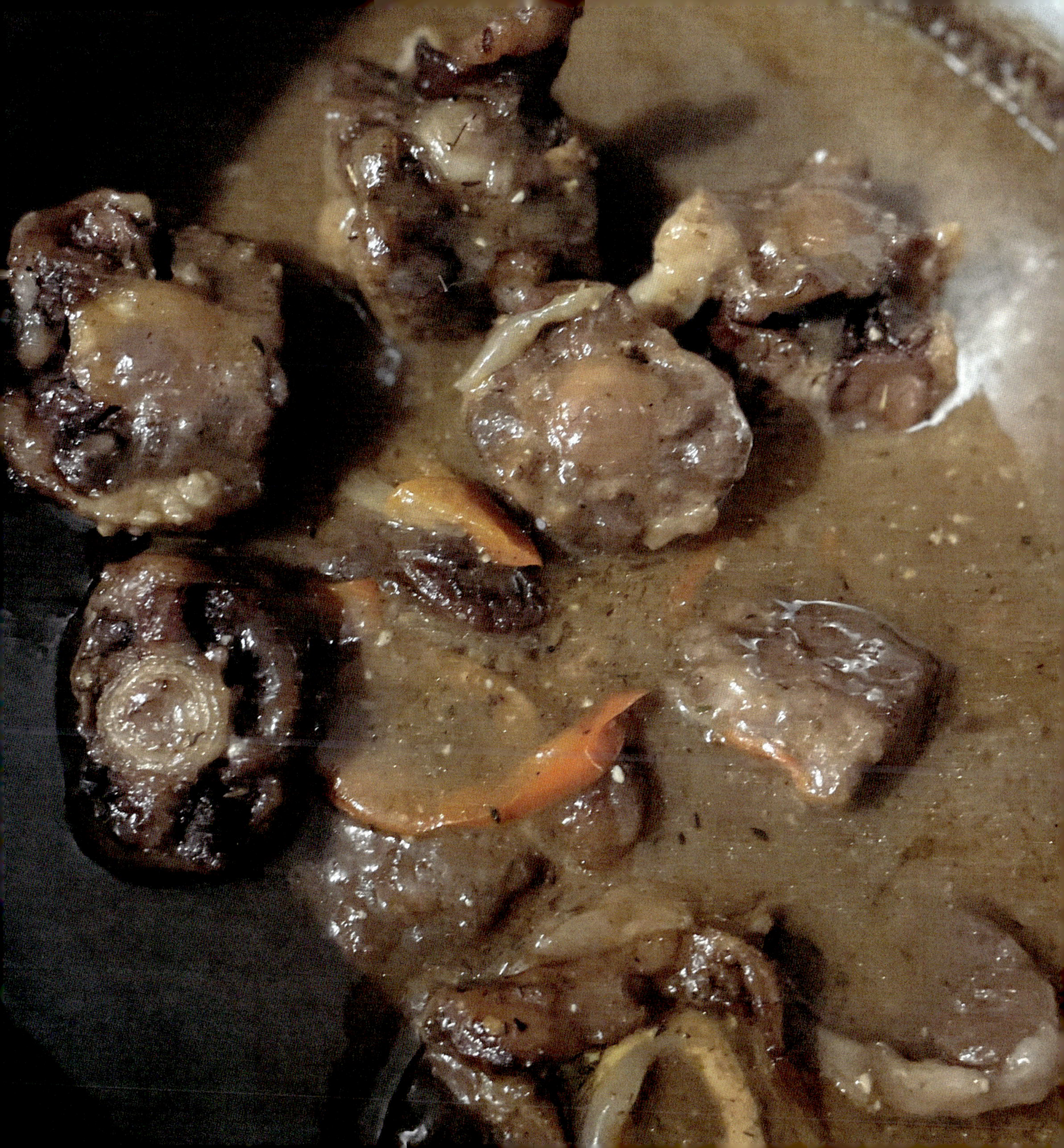

Ingredients

Serves: 4-6

1 - 2 lb. Oxtails
1 yellow onion
1 green bell pepper
1 red bell pepper
1 cup cooked chopped bacon
1 garlic bulb(peel throw them in whole
1/2 cup chopped Italian parsley
2 tablespoon garlic powder
1 teaspoon basil (dry)
1 teaspoon thyme (dry)
1 teaspoon salt (I went easy)
1 teaspoon black pepper
1 stick salted butter
A pinch of cayenne pepper
A pinch of white sugar
Creole Cajun Queen creole seasoning *(use any creole seasoning or order mine on line)*
1 cup white flour
1 cup red wine
1 can beef stock
1-2 cups water
1/2 cup tomato sauce
1 cup green onion
2 cups cooked white rice

Instructions on next page

Instructions

1. I wash and dry my oxtails then coat with olive oil. Season with salt, pepper and garlic powder. Slice your onions and bell peppers, set aside.

2. I chopped up 1 cup bacon fried it down and put them aside. I fried my oxtails down in the bacon grease until brown on all sides, tossed in my onions, garlic, green onions and bell peppers. While my ingredients are all frying together I added my wine, watched the smoke, then added butter, 1 can beef stock, water, tomato sauce and let it simmer all together on a medium heat for about 20 minutes. I make sure my sauce cover my oxtails.

3. Finally, I add in my flour and give it a stir. I add in the rest of my dry seasonings, cover tightly and place in the oven on 350 for 3 hours. I like to sometimes throw in potatoes and carrots (completely up to you) when it's completely tender, top with Italian parsley and serve over rice.

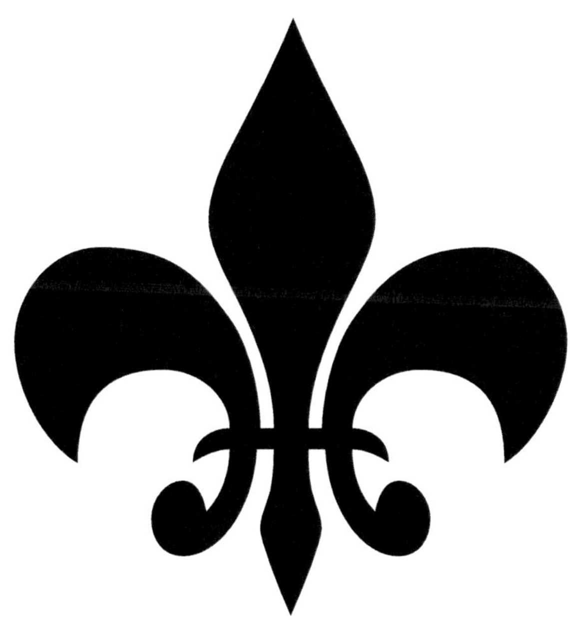

Creole Cajun Queen Bread Pudding

Bread Pudding was a traditional dessert on our table growing up next to the banana pudding or peach cobbler. Sometimes I ate just to get the dessert. In New Orleans French bread doesn't go to waste. Bread Pudding has turned into a delicacy all its own. It's takes a practiced eye and a trained hand to create a delicious bread pudding. You see on first look it just seems like left overs being repurposed. But to a wise and knowledgeable Cajun Chef it's anything but.

First off it takes the finest ingredients to create a first class Bread Pudding. Even down to the bread. Often excess bread was baked for the purpose of using it to prepare this community favorite. Many a meal was rushed to be eaten, just so they could get to that yummy bread pudding. When you see it on the table, realize lots of love, care and expectations went into creating it

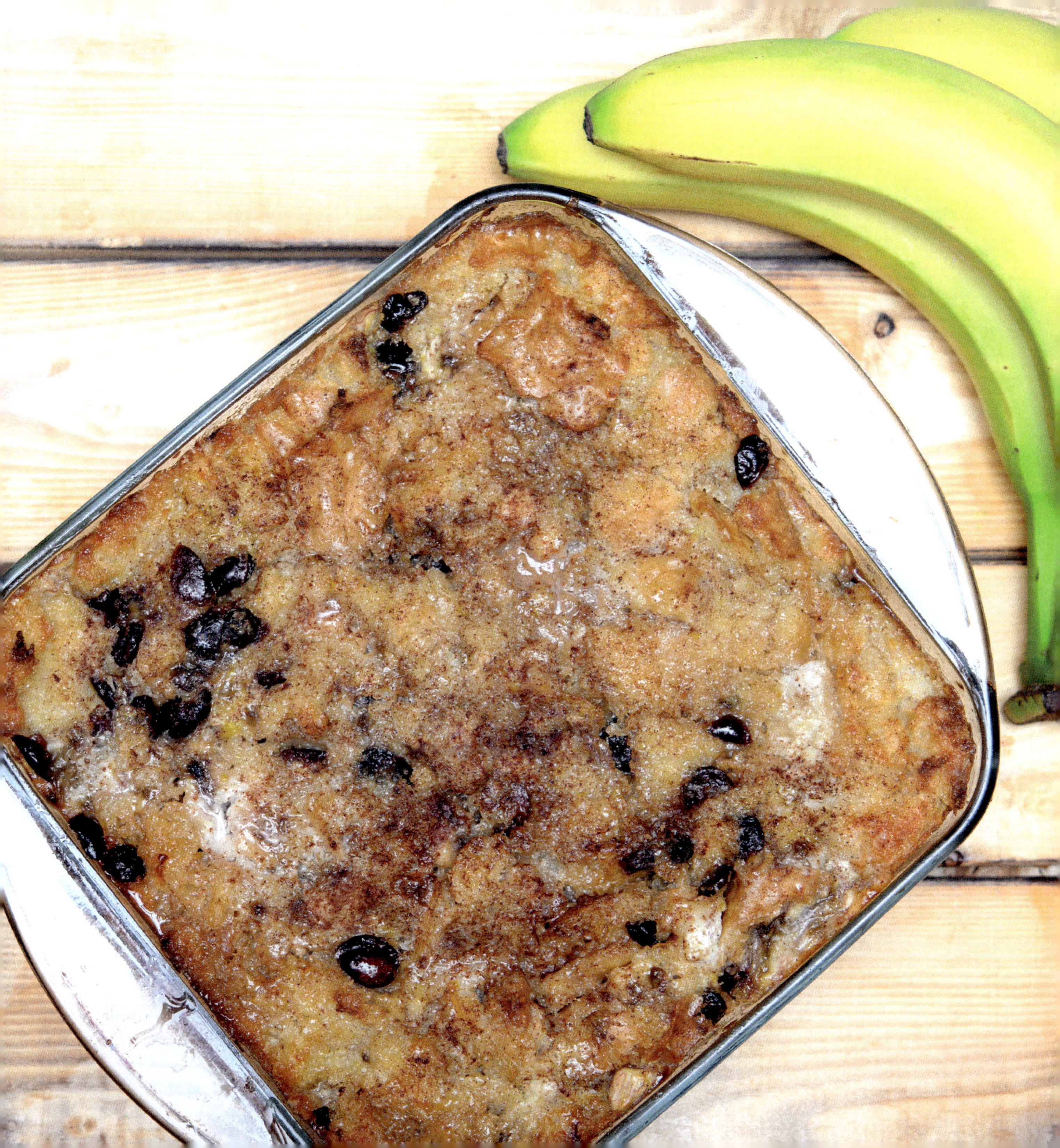

Ingredients

Serves: 4-6

1 French bread loaf
1 cup white sugar
1 cup brown sugar
2 bananas diced up
1/2 cup caramel
1teaspoon vanilla
1 teaspoon cinnamon
1 stick salted butter
1-2 cans cream
1 cup raisins

Rum sauce:

1/2 can condensed milk
1 tablespoon rum
1 teaspoon vanilla extract
1/2 stick butter

Instructions

Rum sauce instructions:

In a small sauce pan stir your condensed milk, rum, butter and vanilla slowly on a low heat until the mixture is blended thick.

(continued on next page)

Instructions (continued)

1. Pull apart your French bread into chunk size pieces. Place pieces in a 9" greased square pan.

2. Mix in bowl 5 eggs, try 1 can of cream first, and add both sugars, cinnamon, vanilla, bananas, raisins and caramel mixing thoroughly.

3. Pour mixture over the bread soaking each piece. Allow to soak for about 5 minutes not leaving the bread soggy enough to break down the bread into crumbs. I melt the butter using 1/2 to pour over the pudding before I Bake in the oven on 350 for 50 minutes. After it is baked I check to make sure the middle is soft but firm and drizzle the rum sauce on top and serve.

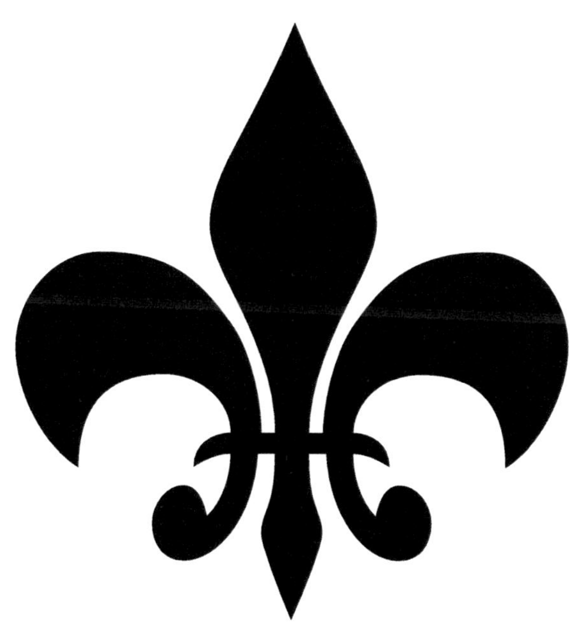

Creole Cajun Queen Peach Cobbler

Peach cobbler is one of my favorite desserts.
I loved going from house to house tasting the
different ways family and friends made it.
The fight was always about crust or cobbler mix.
I love crust!!!

So in this case for me the crust wins.

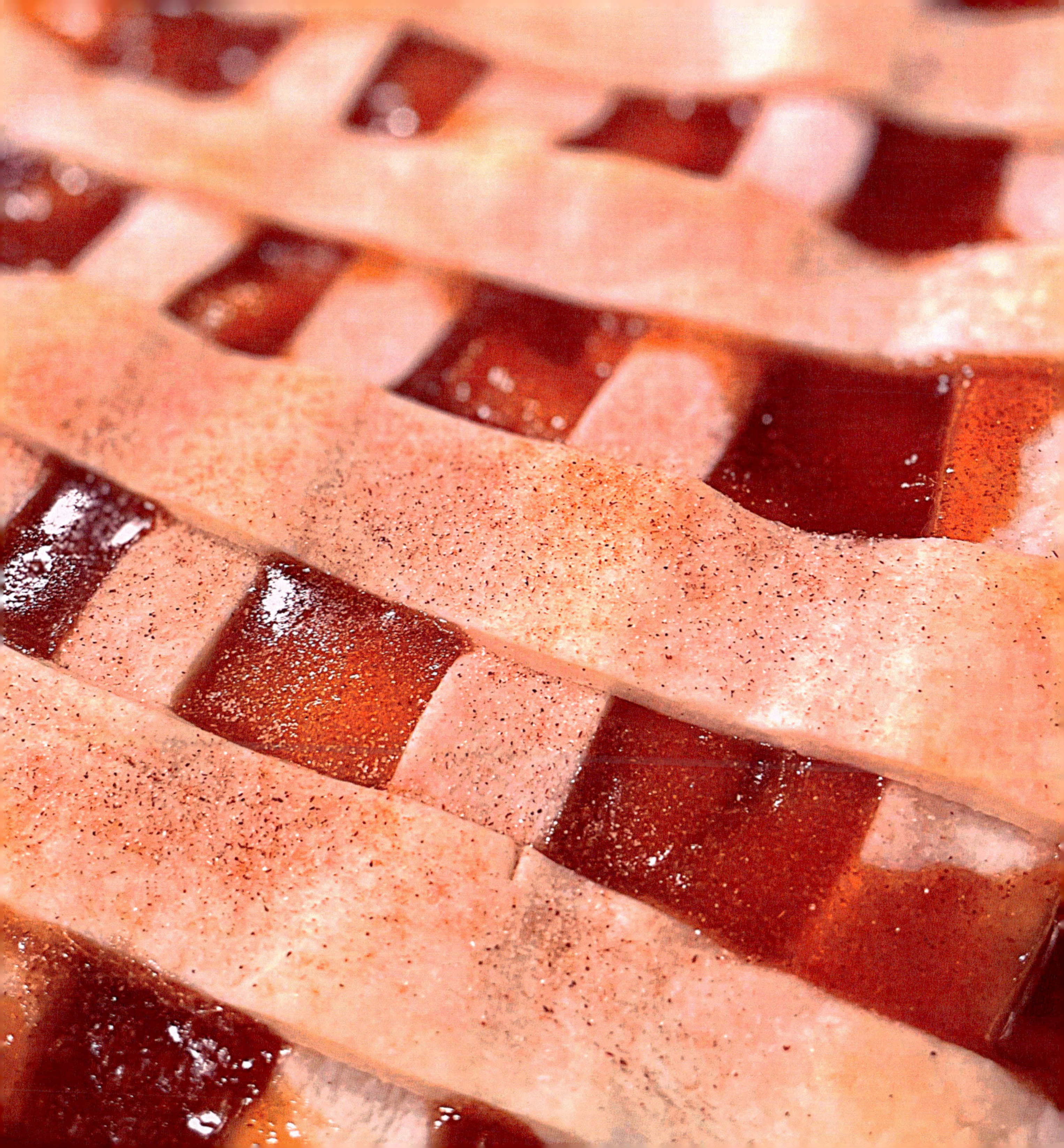

Ingredients

Serves: 4-6

2 cans of 29oz slice peaches in heavy syrup
2 cups white sugar
1 stick salted butter
1 tablespoon vanilla extract
1/2 cup caramel
1/2 teaspoon lemon juice
1 teaspoon cinnamon
1cup brown sugar
1-2 tablespoon corn starch for thickening.
1 egg and a little water for egg wash.

Pie crust:
2 1/2. Cups All purpose white flour
2 Sticks Salted butter
1 tablespoon White sugar
5-7 tablespoon Ice Water
(A store brought pie crust is also just as good).
1/2 stick butter

Instructions

1. If you are making your pie crust, in a bowl add your flour, cubed butter, sugar in a food processor. Little by little add in your ice water to add moist to your dough.

2. Shake a little flour on your clean counter, scoop the dough out break it into two pieces and roll each pieces in a ball. Wrap in plastic and chill for 1 hour.

3. In a medium heavy sauce pot add in your peaches, both sugars,vanilla, lemon juice , cinnamon and stick of butter on a low-medium heat stirring. Allow the sauce to boil and add the caramel while on a low boil.

(continued on next page)

Instructions (continued)

4. In a small bowl mix 2 tablespoons of cornstarch and water into a pasty mix, add in the cornstarch and mix evenly. Cover your pot with a lid lower the heat and allow the sauce to thicken. Once the sauce is thick turn off your heat.

5. Take out both your dough balls and roll one out to fit a greased pie dish. The second dough ball roll out and cut into long strips and set aside. Brush your dough in your dish with egg wash and bake in the oven until the crust is lightly brown. In your browned crust add in your peach mixture.

6. Take your dough strips and lay them 1 inch apart long ways and lay some strips 1 inch apart short ways in another direction across your first strips. Brush with egg wash , bake in the oven on 350 for 25 minutes or until the crust is golden brown. Cool and eat.

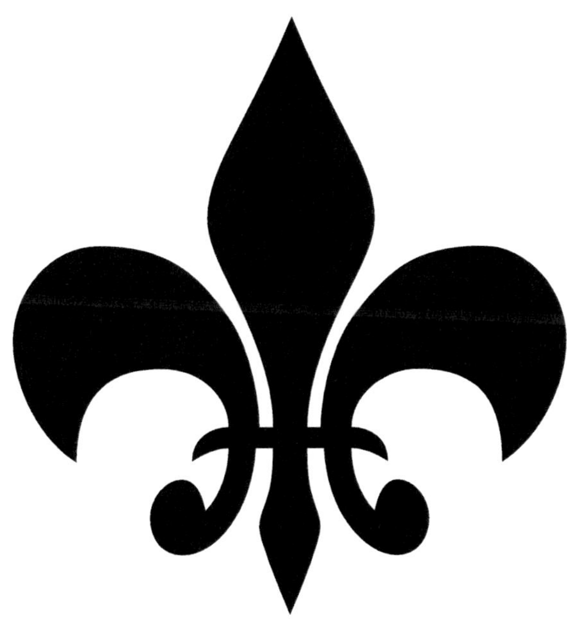

Creole Cajun Queen Shrimp or Crawfish Etouffee'

This dish takes me back to my Sister Penny's debutant ball days. I was 9 years old and going to this ball was amazing in my eyes. The tables were set up so beautiful and you can go from table to table and see what kind of food each table had and of course we threw down as always with Shrimp or Crawfish 'Etouffée, chicken and spaghetti Mac and cheese.

This was also my brother Mark's favorite dish . He moved to California and realized I can cook lol, and would visit asking for this dish.

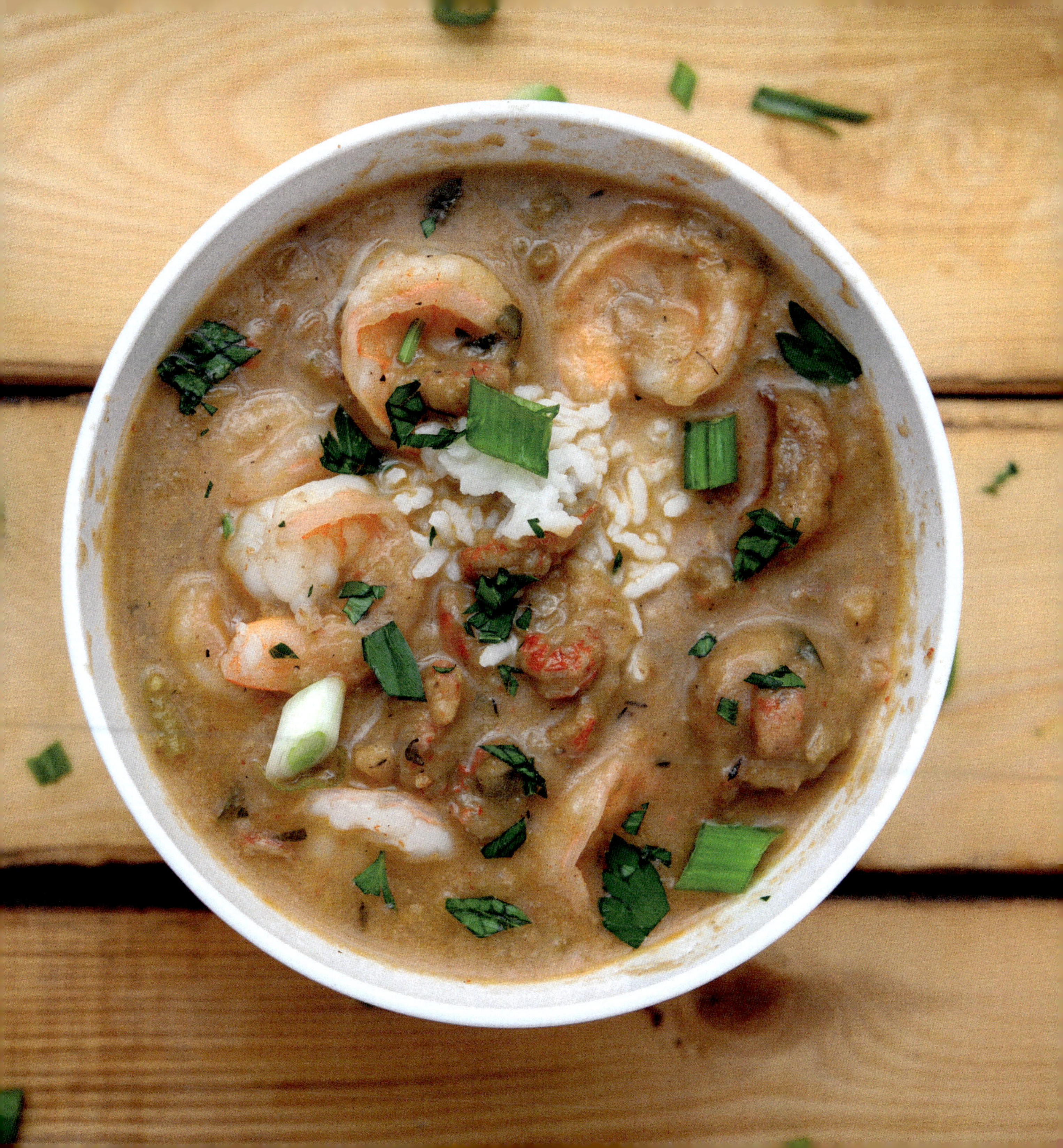

Ingredients

Serves: 4-6

1 yellow onion
1/2 green bell pepper
1/2 red bell pepper
1 pound of clean deveined large shrimp or 1 pack of crawfish
4 cloves of chopped garlic
1/2 cup of celery
1/2 cup of tomato sauce or you can use diced tomatoes
1/2 teaspoon of thyme
1 bay leaf
2 tablespoons of bacon grease
1 tablespoon of chop green onions
1/2 teaspoon chop Italian parsley
1 stick of salted butter
2 cups of chicken broth
1/4 teaspoon of crab boil
1/2 teaspoon of basil
1 tablespoon creole Cajun Queen creole seasoning *(use any creole seasoning or order mine on line)*
1 tablespoon of garlic powder
1/2 teaspoon of salt
1/2 teaspoon black pepper
2 tablespoon white flour
2 cup cooked white rice

Instructions on next Page

Instructions

1. Dice your onions, garlic,bell peppers and celery. Next in a cast iron on metal pot melt your butter and bacon grease down getting it really hot blending together on a medium heat. If you are using crawfish in a package drain and wash lightly.set your cleaned shrimp with crawfish aside.Add in your flour and stir until your roux starts to lightly brown.

2. Add your bell pepper, onions ,celery and fry down in the pot stirring in with the roux mix evenly. Next toss in the shrimp and cook until it's pink, add in your dry seasoning , tomato sauce,chicken stock and crawfish then mix together on a medium heat.

3. Last let it bubble and get a little thicker. Turn off your heat serve over rice garnish with green onions and parsley.

Bon appetite!

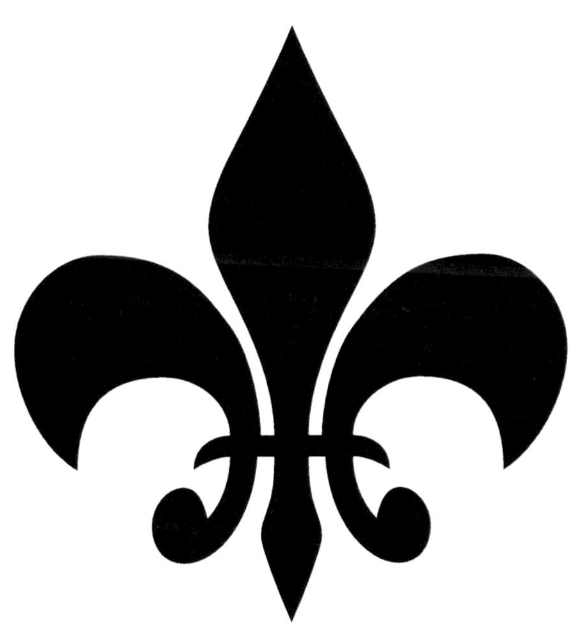

Creole Cajun Queen Crawfish Pasta

Crawfish pasta reminds me of the good times I had at many festivals. Even though my family can cook this dish at home it was always a treat to go out to the jazz festival or French Quarter festival to taste other's pasta and act like a tourist.

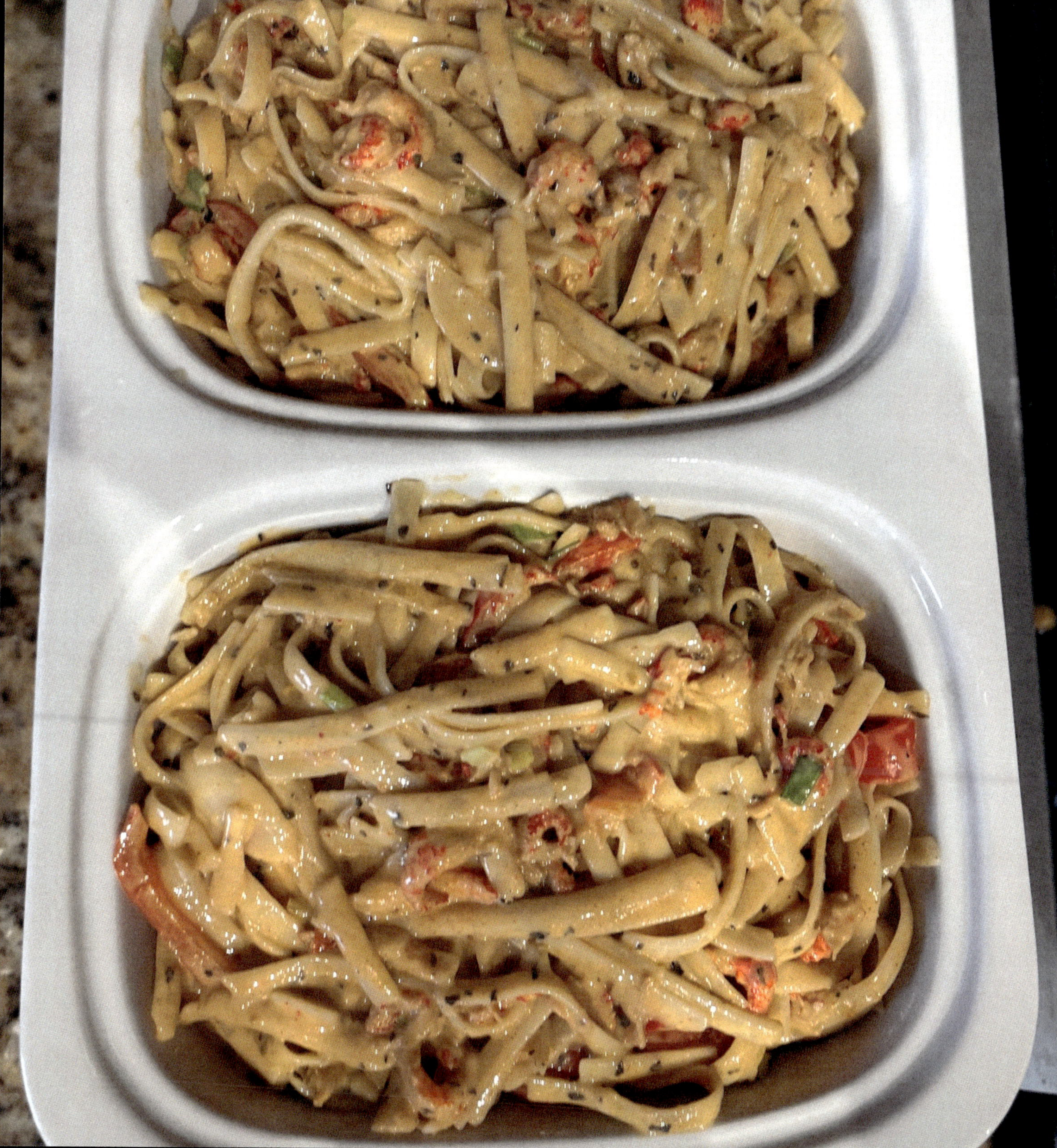

Ingredients

Serves: 4

1 pack crawfish tails or 1 pound fresh crawfish tails.
1 yellow onion
1 red bell pepper
1 tablespoon crushed garlic
1 tablespoon Italian parsley
Creole Cajun Queen Creole seasoning *(use any creole seasoning or order mine on line)*
1 tablespoon garlic powder
1 cup mild cheddar cheese
1 cup mozzarella cheese
1 cup American cheese
1 teaspoon white sugar
1 pinch cayenne pepper
1 tablespoon dry basil
1 stick of butter
1 stick of margarin
1 can of cream
1 pack fettuccine pasta

Instructions

1. Drain/ lightly wash your crawfish tails or if fresh use as is. Slice or chop your onions, bell peppers and set aside.

2. Boil your pasta until firm but soft. Drain,wash , olive oil it and set aside.

3. In a heavy metal pan heat up your butter and margarin on a medium heat. Sauté your onions and bell peppers until soft.

4. Add in your crawfish tails, crushed garlic and all of the dry seasonings mixing together.

(continued on next page)

Instructions (continued)

5. Next add in 1 can cream to your crawfish mix and stir. Toss in all your cheese. Mix on a low fire until your sauce mix starts to thicken.cut your heat.

6. Pour your crawfish cheese sauce over your pasta and mix evenly. Toss in your parsley. Add more salt, garlic, basil or cayenne pepper to taste if needed. Plate, serve and enjoy.

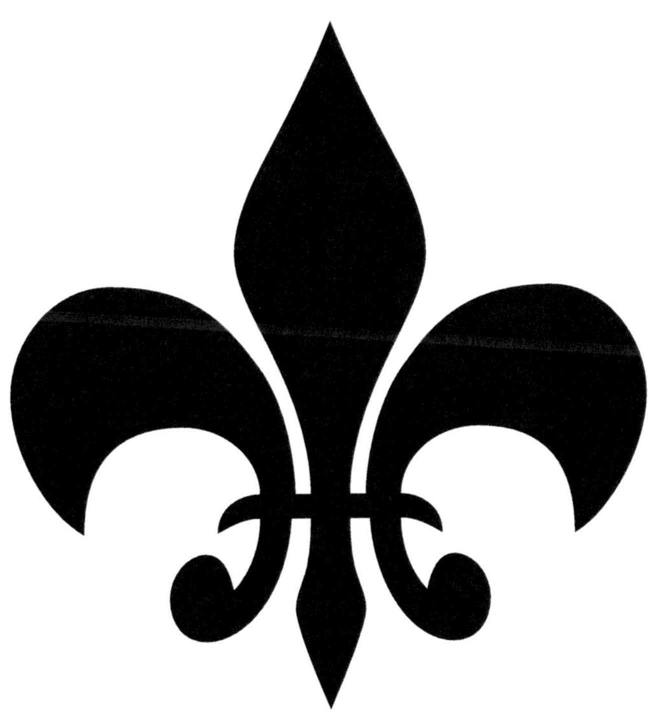

Creole Cajun Queen Chicken and Andouille Sausage Over Rice

In New Orleans gravy and rice was your every day go
to meal with what ever meat your household could afford.
I remember my mom leaving Greater St Stephens church
and right at the corner bus stop she would stop in at the
chicken mart and pick up chicken smoked sausage.
I know what you are all thinking? What is she cooking?
Well let me tell you a, darn good
Sunday meal that stretches.
Lol

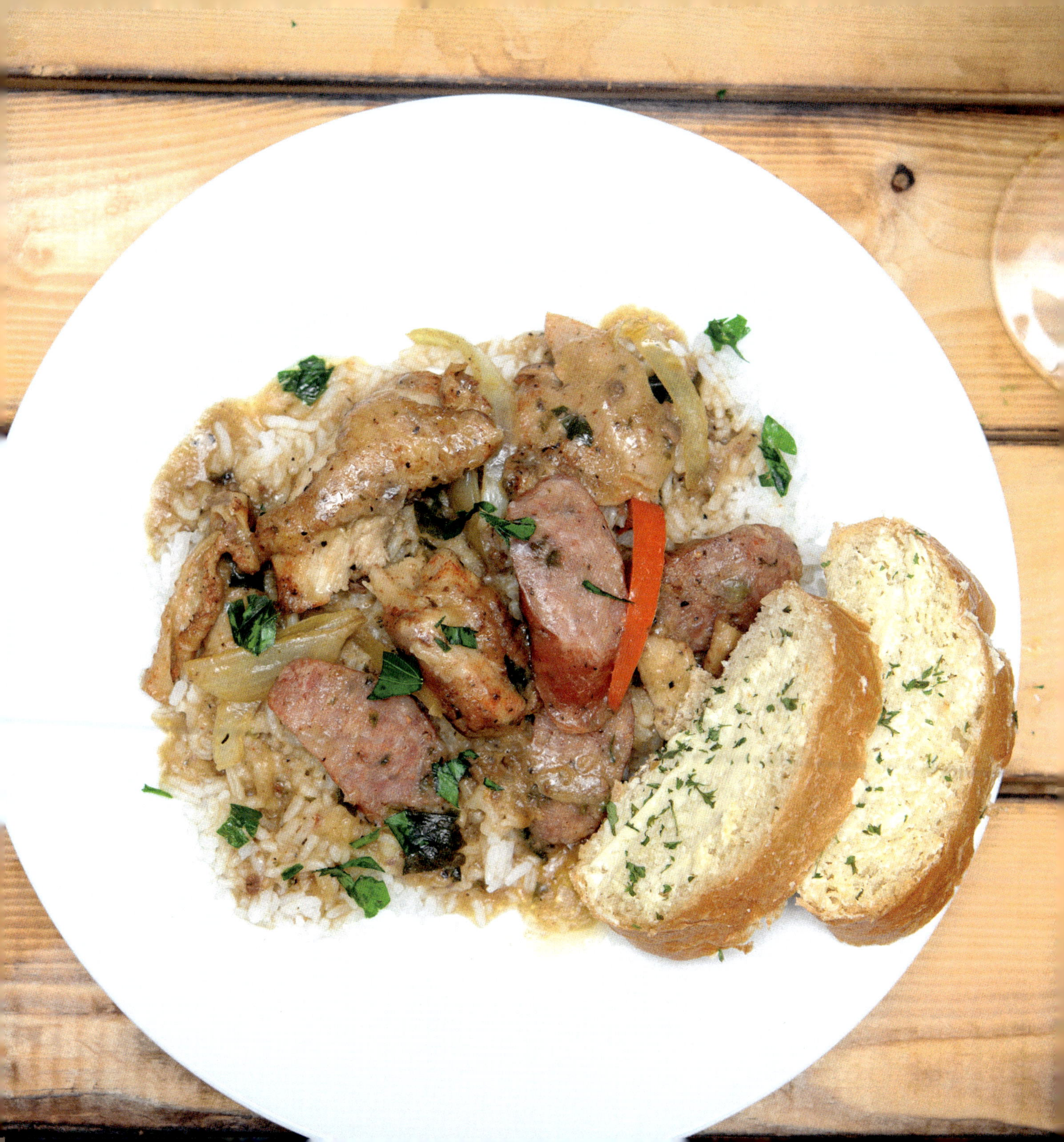

Ingredients

Serves: 4

4 Chicken thighs with the skin on(chicken breast optional)
1 pound andouille sausage
2 cups cooked long grain white rice
1 yellow onion
1 green bell pepper
1 celery stem
1 cup all purpose flour
4 tablespoon bacon grease
1/2 teaspoon salt
1 teaspoon black pepper
1 tablespoon garlic powder
1 tablespoon onion powder
1 tablespoon Creole Cajun Queen creole seasoning *(use any creole seasoning or order mine on line)*
1 tablespoon parsley (fresh or dry)
1/2 cup green onion
2 cups water

Instructions

1. Wash , clean cutting fat off of your chicken thighs and pat dry. Salt and pepper your thighs,Slice your andouille sausage. Chop up your onions, bell pepper and celery (trinity) .

2. In a cast iron or metal pot heat up your bacon grease. To check if the oil is hot, I stand a wooden cooking spoon in the oil and once it bubbles around the spoon you are good to go.

3. Start frying your thighs skin down first until the skin crisp up on a medium heat .(about 4minutes)then flip over cooking for 4 minutes. Remove the chicken to the side.

(continued on next page)

Instructions (continued)

4. In the same grease sauté your trinity until it's soft . Add in your sausage fry and mix together browning the sausage. Remove your mix from the pot using a spoon with wholes to leave your remaining oil in your pot.

5. Add in your flour , cut your heat to low stirring/ mixing together with your oil. Do a slow stir while making sure your flour is even and browning.

6. Once your roux is a cinnamon brown add your garlic powder, onion powder, creole seasoning,sausage and trinity mix in and stir together. Add 2 cups of water then stir until everything is smooth.

7. Add your thighs back into your pot . Cover, turn heat back up to medium and cook / simmer for 1 hour. Serve over a bed of rice and garnish with green onions.

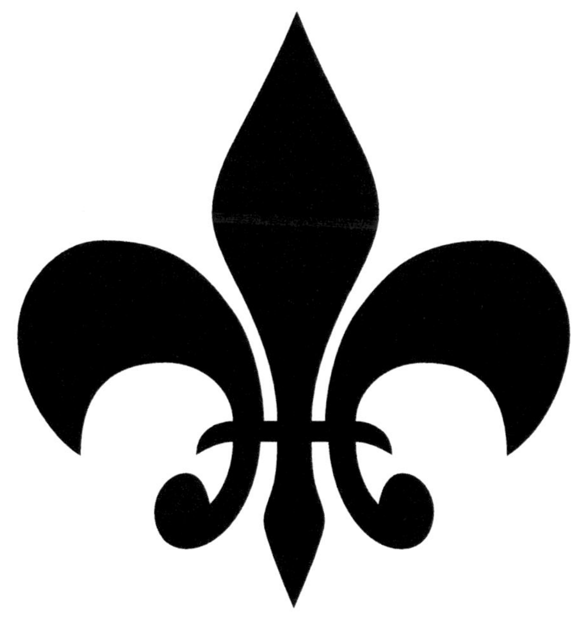

Creole Cajun Queen Blackened Catfish Alfredo Over Pasta

I totally started feeling myself when I started cooking this dish. I can tell you pan searing was a task for me and using too much oil or not enough oil drove me crazy. My Aunts were my taste testers. A lot of my family history was given to me by my Aunts sitting on the sofa as I tested out recipes, as they are reminded of who I cook like in the family. Aunties are just as wonderful as Mothers, they are your secret cheerleaders.

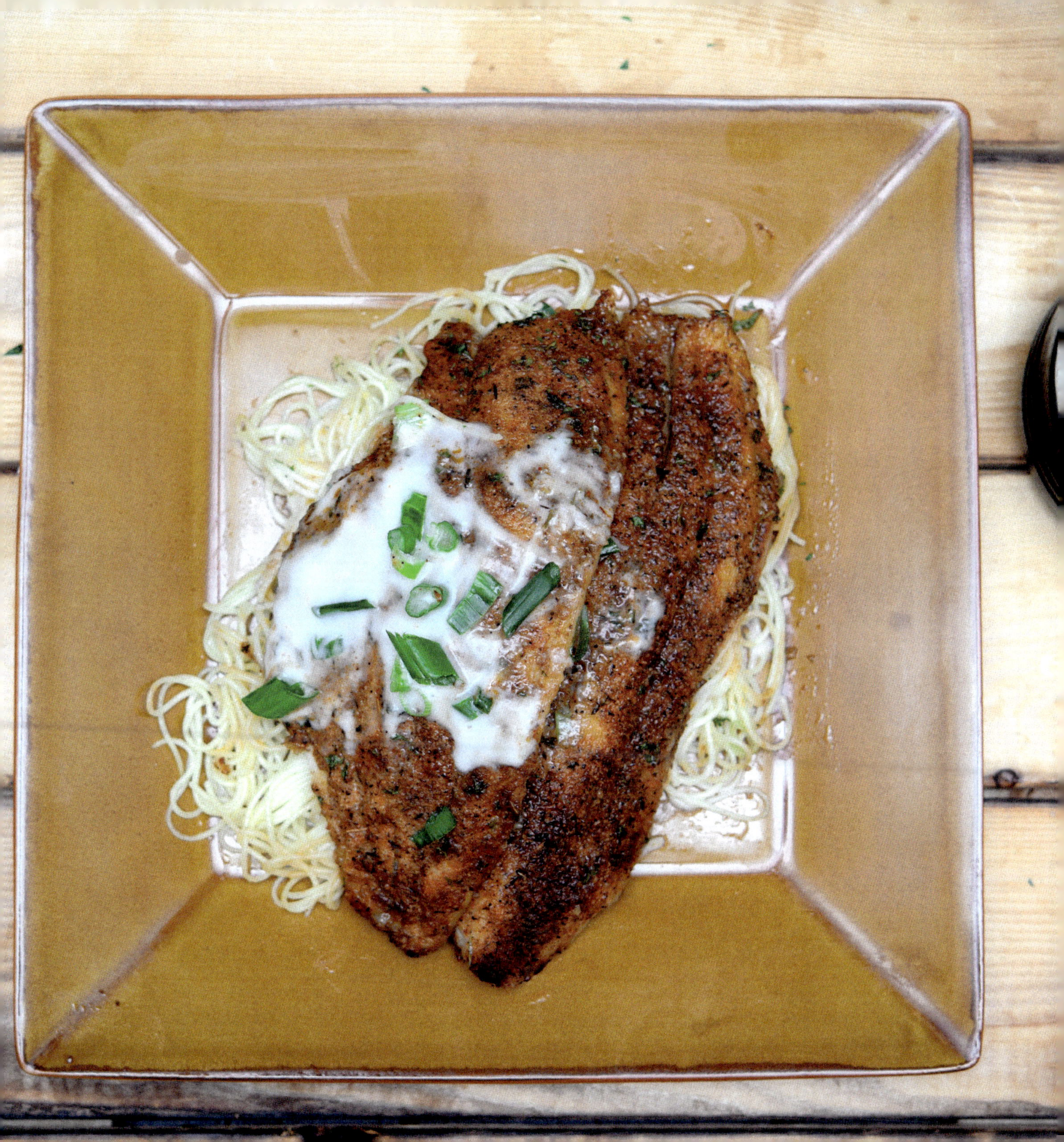

Ingredients

Serves: 2

2 Catfish Fillets
1 teaspoon black garlic powder
1/2 Creole Cajun Queen Creole Seasoning *(use any creole seasoning or order mine on line)*
1/4 teaspoon smoked paprika
1 can of cream
1 stick margarin
1 cup chicken broth
1 cup white American cheese
1 cup shredded Parmesan cheese
1 tablespoon garlic powder
1 pack 12oz boiled Angel hair pasta
1 cup green onion
1/2 cup olive oil
1/2teaspoon white sugar
1 pinch cayenne pepper

Instructions

1. Season your catfish fillets with black garlic powder, smoked paprika and creole seasoning. Heat up oil in a heavy metal frying pan on medium to high heat.

2. Once the grease is hot pan sear (fry)your fish on each side for 3 minutes . (This fish can also be baked in the oven at 350 for 20 minutes).set aside

(continued on next page)

Instructions (continued)

3. Plate your pasta on a plate. Ladle a little of Alfredo sauce on your pasta then lay your fish on top of your pasta and add another Ladle of Alfredo sauce on your fish then garnish with green onions and ooh wee! Sha' let's eat!

Alfredo Sauce: In a sauce pan heat your butter, cream,chicken broth on low to medium heat. Add in both your cheese more garlic powder,Creole Seasoning, cayenne pepper and sugar. Whisk until your sauce is smooth and creamy . Cut your fire.

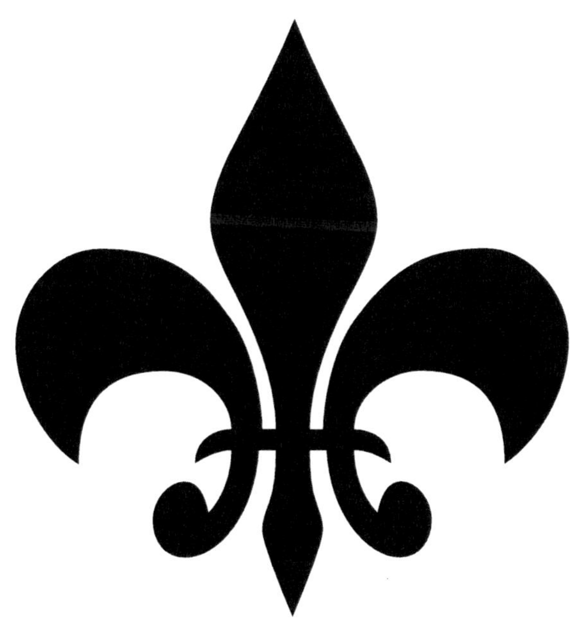

Potato salad

Who made the Potato Salad???

Is the buzzing question when it's served at a New Orleans table. You always have this one sister lol, she's going to kill me, cousin or aunt that wants to volunteer to make potato salad and it's off point. Potato salad is served as a side no matter what we cook.

If you're cooking gumbo?
Potato salad, fried chicken or fish?
Potato salad ,even with a rice dish?
Yesss !Potato salad! You get the picture...

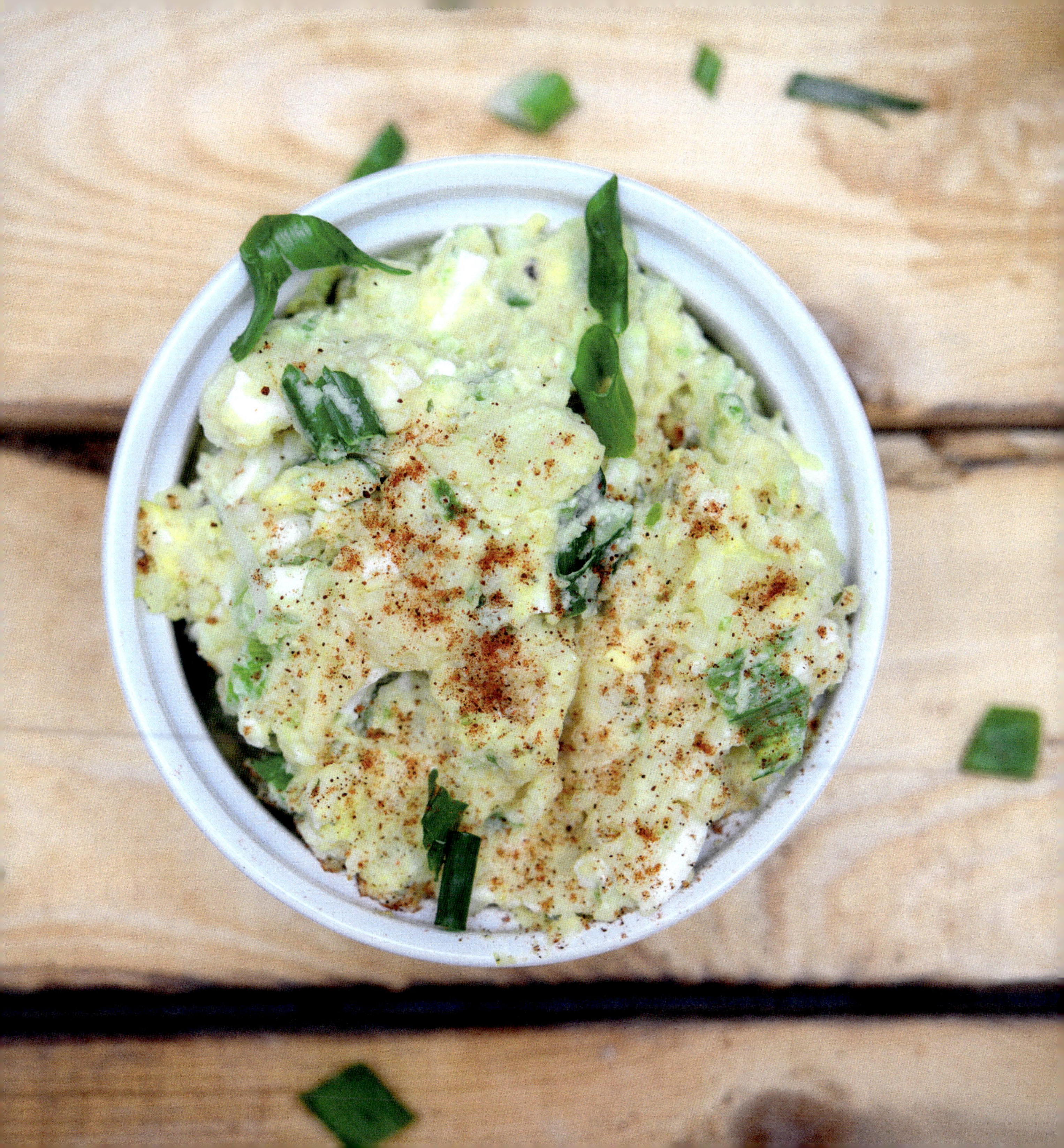

Ingredients

Serves: 4-6

6 -large russet potatoes (sometime I use the red potatoes from my crawfish boil)
12 boiled eggs- I use a lot of eggs
1 yellow onion
1 green bell pepper
1 celery stem
1 cup green onion
1 tablespoon Italian parsley chopped
1 teaspoon powder crab boil (for boiling the potatoes if I don't use the already boiled ones from boils)
1/2 teaspoon Creole Cajun Queen Creole seasoning *(any would do but you can order mine online)*
1/2 teaspoon black pepper
1 tablespoon onion powder
1 tablespoon mustard
2 -3 tablespoon mayonnaise (I use Blue Plate mayonnaise)
1 tablespoon sweet relish
Salt to taste

Instructions

1. I first cut my potatoes in half, fill my pot with water covering the potatoes and sprinkle in my crab boil then boil for about an hour or until the potatoes are firm but soft. Boil your eggs with your potatoes and pull them out first.(8-10 minutes on the eggs)

2. Next, I chop my trinity up(bell pepper, celery and onion) very small. You can use your chopper, chopping is relaxing to me,lol I chop.

3. When your eggs are done cool and peel, then using a egg slicer, slice your eggs up dicing them. Toss in a bowl your seasoning, eggs and chop seasoning.

(continued on next page)

Instructions (continued)

4. Once your potatoes are done, cool , peel the skin off. Mash your potatoes with a potato masher. Stir in your mustard ,mayonnaise and relish mixing all your seasoning and spices together.

5. This last step is important . I make my potato salad smooth yet sometimes a little chunky. Toss in your parsley , mix it in and salt to taste.

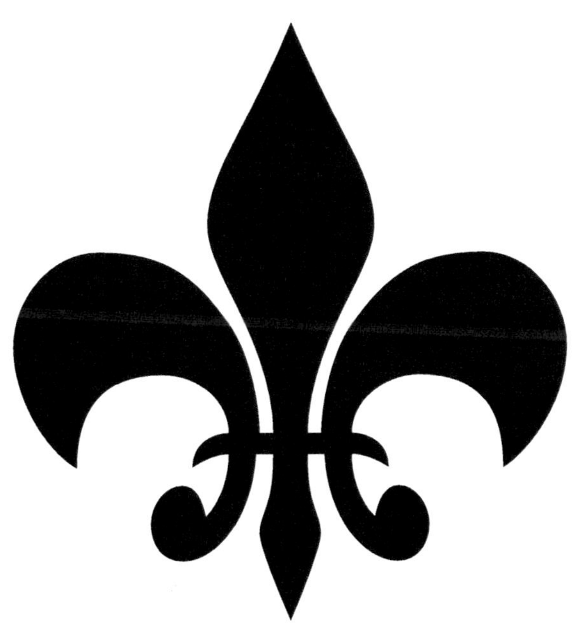

Creole Cajun Queen Gumbo

Gumbo always brings me back to that shot gun house on Jeanette street sitting at that green kitchen table watching my mom separate each ingredient for her gumbo. Standing at her tiny gas stove for hours getting her roux just right gives me some of my best childhood memories. I could never understand why her gumbo was never rushed or why it took so many hours back then. As I have grown and began to love making this dish I now feel the joy, peace and love that was in this gumbo pot. Gumbo has bought my family together, gave us great time spent and joy. My Mom has passed and every time I begin making gumbo I can't help to think she is looking down smiling proud of me. I took care of my mom in her old age and every birthday I would ask my mom what do you want me to cook for your birthday and she would say gumbo. So you see I love cooking but my mom is my true inspiration behind this authentic dish.

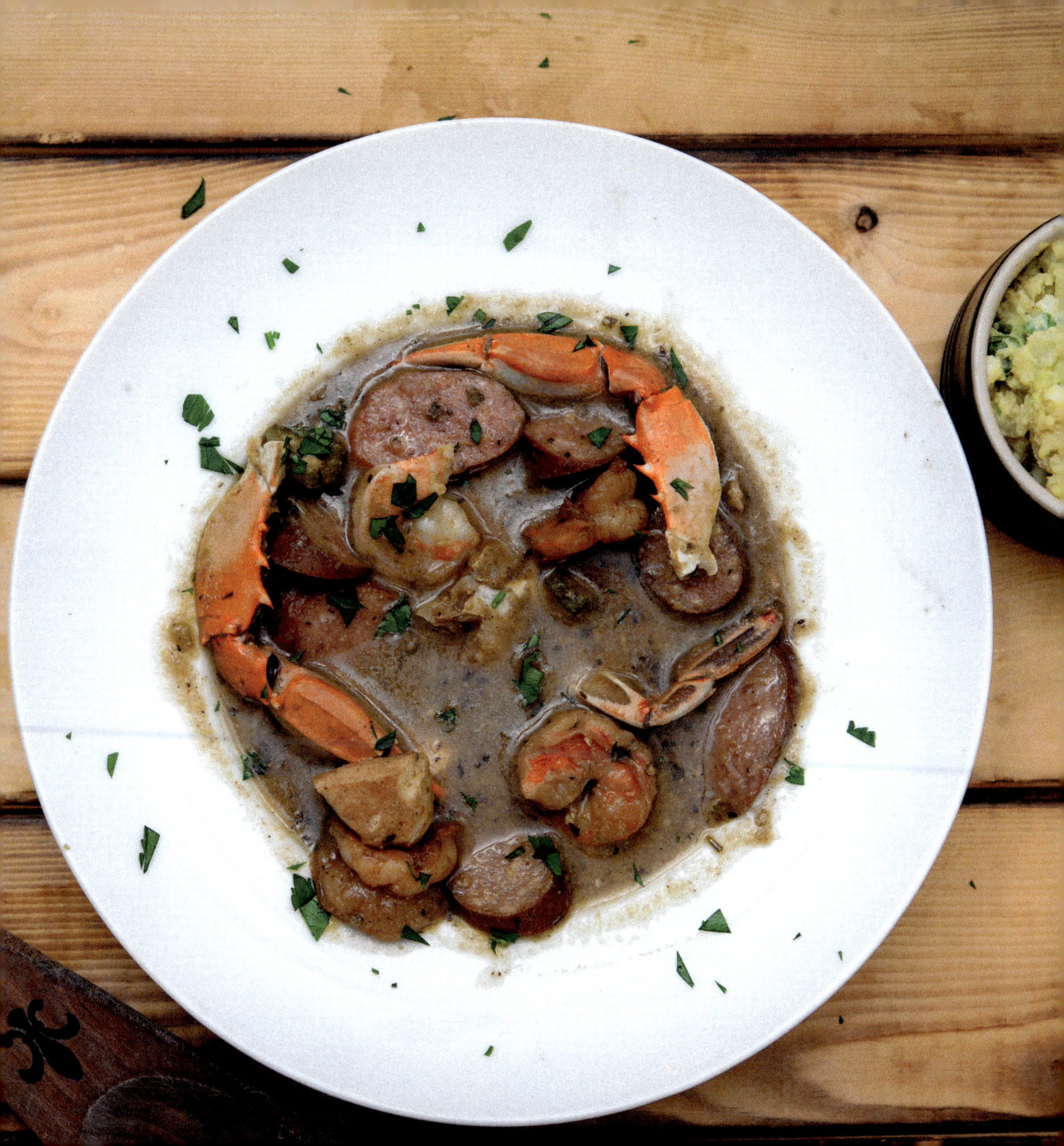

Ingredients

Serves: 6-10

Chicken breast cut in chunks(In New Orleans we use chicken wing parts
4 chicken thighs with the skin on to boil for stock
Double D smoke sausage
(Any smoke sausage will do)
1 lb peeled,cleaned and deveined large shrimp (save the shrimp heads to boil for stock)
3 cleaned , split in 2 blue crabs
1 small pack chicken gizzards (I only use to boil for the broth)
3 cups chicken broth
2 cups shrimp stock
1 cup gizzard liquids
2 yellow onions diced
2 green bell peppers diced
4 celery stems
3 cups fresh sliced okra
4 celery stems diced
4 garlic cloves
2 tablespoon garlic powder
1 tablespoon Creole Cajun Queen creole seasoning (any creole seasoning will do)
1 teaspoon liquid crab boil
1 tablespoon onion powder
2 tablespoon file powder
1 tablespoon Italian seasoning
(yes trust me, lol)
1/2 tablespoon black pepper
2 cups white flour
1/2 cup bacon grease
1 tablespoon liquid crab boil
2 cups cooked white rice
4 bay leaves

Instructions

1. My gumbo process takes 2 days. The day before you cook your gumbo chop up your trinity (onions,bell pepper and celery) slice your smoke sausage and leave covered in fridge over night.

2. The day of cooking I boil my gizzards, chicken thighs and shrimp heads together in crab boil and a shake of garlic powder. I used to do it separately but realized all the juices are going in the same pot. Boil for a good hour. Strain and drain your juice into your big metal gumbo pot.

3. Cut up your chicken breast into chunks season with salt and pepper and cook on a medium heat. You will see your juices also from your breast. Throw that juicy in also. Don't cook it all the way through it will finish in your gumbo. Set aside.

4. In in a big heavy metal Stock pot , heat up your bacon grease . Use the end of a wooden spoon to check to see if your grease is hot. (if the grease bubbles around the stick then it's ready) begin adding your flour and stir until you get a nice peanut butter color or little darker for your roux . I like darker. (Attention!!!! Don't leave your roux! Stand there and keep stirring on a low to medium heat until you get the right color) don't rush your roux!!! Put on some music and chill. Lol. Once your roux has the dark pasty consistency and your kitchen is smoking haha add in your trinity and mix in evenly.

5. At this point your stocks are ready. combine all of your stock in your big gumbo pot mixing it with your roux and trinity seasoning evenly. Add in your chicken breast, smoke sausage and okra. Bring to a boil for about 45 minutes on a medium heat. Add in all of your dry seasoning and stir.

6. After boiling for 45 minutes, throw in your shrimp and blue crabs. Cook , covered for 20 minutes more. Salt and spice up to taste. I always keep a separate cup of shrimp stock on the side. Gumbo is a taste to season dish for me. Serve over rice and enjoy.

Made in the USA
Middletown, DE
03 October 2024

61988192R00064